The Yogic Writer

The Yogic Writer

Uniting Breath, Body, and Page

Jennifer Sinor

BLOOMSBURY ACADEMIC
LONDON • NEW YORK • OXFORD • NEW DELHI • SYDNEY

BLOOMSBURY ACADEMIC
Bloomsbury Publishing Plc
50 Bedford Square, London, WC1B 3DP, UK
1385 Broadway, New York, NY 10018, USA
29 Earlsfort Terrace, Dublin 2, Ireland

BLOOMSBURY, BLOOMSBURY ACADEMIC and the Diana logo are
trademarks of Bloomsbury Publishing Plc

First published in Great Britain 2024

Copyright © Jennifer Sinor, 2024

Jennifer Sinor has asserted her right under the Copyright,
Designs and Patents Act, 1988, to be identified as author of this work.

For legal purposes the acknowledgments on p. xiv constitute an
extension of this copyright page.

Cover design by Rebecca Heselton
Cover image © Aziz Fatima07/ Shutterstock

All rights reserved. No part of this publication may be reproduced or transmitted
in any form or by any means, electronic or mechanical, including photocopying,
recording, or any information storage or retrieval system, without prior
permission in writing from the publishers.

Bloomsbury Publishing Plc does not have any control over, or responsibility for, any
third-party websites referred to or in this book. All internet addresses given in this
book were correct at the time of going to press. The author and publisher regret
any inconvenience caused if addresses have changed or sites have ceased to
exist but can accept no responsibility for any such changes.

The author and publisher gratefully acknowledge the permission granted to reproduce
copyrighted material in this book. The third party copyrighted material displayed in the
pages of this book is done so on the basis of fair use for the purposes of teaching,
criticism, scholarship or research only in accordance with international copyright laws,
and is not intended to infringe upon the ownership rights of the original owners.

A version of the chapter "Breathing to Write" first appeared in *The Writer's Chronicle* under
the same name. Parts of "Finding Form" first appeared in *The Writer's* Chronicle as "Brief
But True." Parts of "Crafting Voices" was first published as "Crafting Voice" in *The Rose Metal
Press Field Guide to Writing Flash Nonfiction: Advice and Essential Exercises from Respected
Writers, Editors, and Teachers,* edited by Dinty W. Moore, Rose Metal Press, 2012.

A catalogue record for this book is available from the British Library.
A catalog record for this book is available from the Library of Congress.

ISBN: HB: 978-1-3503-7195-8
PB: 978-1-3503-7196-5
ePDF: 978-1-3503-7197-2
eBook: 978-1-3503-7198-9

Typeset by Integra Software Services Pvt. Ltd.

To find out more about our authors and books visit www.bloomsbury.com
and sign up for our newsletters.

For my teachers

What the rain can do for a well, so can the language from an illumined heart.

—HAFIZ

CONTENTS

Acknowledgments xiv

Introduction: The Sky Inside 1

Part One Beginnings—*Pūraka*

1 Writing with the Whole Body 9
   The sheaths of the yogic body

2 Born to Write 13
   Not seeking validation from others

3 Set Your Goats to Roam 16
   Art as the externalization of the internal

4 Breathing to Write 19
   Breath practice: intentional breathing

5 Effortless Effort 23
   Allowing your attention to be called to what you love

6 Form the Circle and Step Inside 26
   Creating a sacred writing space

7 Don't Wait for Cadaver Gums 29
   Importance of daily practice

8 The Portable Altar 32
   Flexibility in your practice

9 Casting Language 35
   Keeping a writing notebook

10 X Always Marks the Spot 39
    Writing prompt: mapping childhood
11 Picture This 42
    Writing prompt: writing from a photo
12 I'll Never 44
    Writing prompt: writing into the difficult
13 Inhale the Stars 47
    Breath practice: focus on inhalation
14 Fiction Doesn't Exist 49
    Finding compassion for yourself
15 On Fire 52
    Writing prompt: sparking intuition
16 Archives Aren't for the Dead 55
    Writing from primary materials
17 Trust the Treasure 58
    Staying with a memory
18 No One Blames the Baby 62
    The importance of becoming
19 The Spellwork of Others 65
    The practice of daily reading
20 Writer's Eyes 68
    Seeing as reception
21 The Muse Is a Myth 71
    The labor of craft

Part Two Fullness—*Āntara Kumbhaka*

22 Fullness 77
    Breath practice: retention at the top of the inhalation
23 Dander and Fluff 80
    Start small

CONTENTS

24 Everyone Gets Naked in a Scene 83
    Writing scenes
25 Designate a Driver 87
    Writing summary
26 There Is No Beethoven 90
    The musing voice
27 Breathing with Caesar 93
    Breath practice: keeping the breath sacred
28 Enter Snake 95
    Significant detail
29 No Dead Grandmothers 98
    Creating characters
30 Whose Line Is It? 102
    Creating dialogue
31 What to Bring to Show and Tell 106
    The power of both showing and telling
32 What Piano? 110
    Pursuing organic metaphors
33 The Body Is Your Swing 114
    Breath practice: somatic movement
34 Creating Our Own Obstacles 118
    The myth of writer's block
35 Research and Laundry 121
    Archival and living research
36 Crafting Voice 125
    Voice is made not discovered
37 It's Not about Cake 129
    Finding deeper subject
38 Drop the Knife 133
    Breath practice: loving kindness

39 The Body, The House 137
    Writing and trauma

40 Finding Form 140
    Linear and nonlinear structure

Part Three Distillation—*Recaka*

41 Winnowing 147
    Breath practice: exhalation

42 See the Wolf 150
    Understanding fundamental attributes

43 Collecting Language 154
    Precise diction

44 Choosing Your Wand 158
    Verbs as energetic channels

45 Heart Holding 162
    Breath practice: holding your own heart

46 Word by Word by Word 165
    Focusing on syntax

47 Taking Refuge 169
    Forming a writing group

48 The Public in Publication 173
    Alternative types of publication

49 Rejection as Protection 176
    How to keep going

Part Four Void—*Bāhya Kumbhaka*

50 Entering the Void 183
    Breath practice: retention at the bottom

51 The Alchemy of Writing 186
   Connections between yoga, alchemy, and writing
52 Surrender Ritual 190

Conclusion 192

Bibliography 194

ACKNOWLEDGMENTS

When asked who her guru is, my dear friend Antra Sinha-Waters, always responds, "Whoever is before me." My teachers have given me so much and are far too many in number to name, but they include the sun, the ocean, and the birds, as well as my students, family, friends, and strangers. Here, I honor my most influential teacher, who happens to also be my husband, Michael Sowder. I would not write, I would not practice, and I would not have found this path or these words without him. He shows me every day what it means to love and serve. I also want to name my gratitude for the yogic path in general and to those who initially came from India to the West to share the power of yoga. I have tried to make myself a worthy student of this ancient practice, but I am aware that I still have much to learn.

Introduction: The Sky Inside

A year or so ago, I was hiking with my husband in Little Cottonwood Canyon above Salt Lake City. Even though it was June 24, Michael's birthday, gray skies, and rain accompanied our every step. Fog obscured the trail, and we became lost, but we kept moving up the mountain toward what we thought could be the home of Cecret Lake, an alpine lake that sits at 9,875 feet. At one point, we ran into fellow travelers who hiked by GPS. Turned out, they were just as lost. We each took separate paths up the slope. Because Michael and I had set out so early, the dawn had only recently breached the high peaks. Most often, we hiked in shadow.

The rains grew earnest, turning to sleet, at the moment we arrived at Cecret Lake. Still, the remote lake was beautiful, with a clarity of water so sharp it almost hurt. We walked the boulder fields around the lake, pointing to the wildflowers—paintbrush, penstemons, lupine—that would, in two weeks or so, carpet the valleys of Albion Basin. For now they gathered in thin bouquets set near rocks with the care of a florist. Rain dimpled the lake, bent the flower stems, slid down our cheeks. Wet and cold, we chose not to linger but instead began the long trek back to a car we had parked outside gates still locked for the season. Anyone who has hiked at that elevation knows that going down is harder than coming up. Our boots slipped on every soaked rock. I wished for a walking stick.

All at once, though, the sky cleared. Arms of sunlight swept across the valley floor, illuminating flower, pine, and path. A residue of rain still fell lightly, drops released from clouds that had already passed.

"This would be the perfect time to see a rainbow," Michael said to me. He walked in front because I always hiked slowly going down.

I looked up at the mix of clouds and sun, each drop of rain prismatic and lit from within. "Oh, it would be so perfect to see a rainbow on your birthday!" I searched the sky in vain, kept turning in all directions, willing a rainbow to arc the sky.

Nothing.

We continued the trek down, meeting a pair of hikers who wore black Hefty garbage bags for rain ponchos. It seemed to be a mother and teenaged child. Their breathing came hard, a mixture of sweat and rain on their foreheads. We came together on the trail.

"Did you see the rainbow?" the woman asked us. She pointed to the sky at our backs.

I turned, saw just blue and cloud. "No," I replied. "Was there one?"

"Oh, yes!" she exclaimed. "It was just beautiful. An entire rainbow, even hints of a double one," she said, checking with her teenager, who nodded in confirmation.

We left the pair and continued down the trail, moving more and more into summer with every step as the wildflowers and temperature increased. The entire way down I complained about the fact that we hadn't seen the rainbow on Michael's birthday. The beauty had been withheld. Michael kept pointing to the flowers, returning me again and again to the color before us, but I perseverated on what we had lost.

"I can't believe we missed it," I said for the tenth time. By now we were close to the car, our clothes dry and the sun shining. I stopped to take a drink from my water bottle.

"But it was still there, Jennifer," Michael responded. "We hiked beneath it the entire time. We just couldn't see it."

That is yoga. The knowledge that all the beauty, all the grace, all the fullness of this world already belongs to you. There is nowhere to go. You have everything you need and have been robbed of nothing. But as my story reveals, that is a hard space, as humans, to occupy. While our wholeness is true in the deepest sense, our everyday experience often arrives cloaked in lack, neglect, and disappointment. We tend to focus on the fact that we missed seeing the rainbow rather than the knowledge that the rainbow didn't miss us.

Our world, especially our Western late capitalist world, operates on a model of scarcity. It insists that we are not rich enough, strong enough, pretty enough, or good enough, and that we must, for the most part, consume more to address the lack. This is not a new story; it is just a perfected story, honed to precision by commercialism, globalism, and social media. Long ago, in the forests outside villages in northern India, the Buddha named the fact that our suffering comes from believing that we do not have enough. We have known about the problem for centuries but cannot seem to escape it. Blame it on evolution and the millions of years that human beings literally faced scarcity, or blame it on the fact that humans have a highly developed brain capable of manufacturing fears and anxieties that have little basis in reality, or don't blame anyone and simply accept it as a truth, but we spend much of our time believing the rainbow is not there. That we have missed it. That it never came. That someone else was given the rainbow instead.

What Is Yoga?

We cannot create art from a space riddled with anxiety and fear. More specifically, we cannot create art from a space that is wallowing in the past or afraid for the future. Anxiety and fear are almost always based on circumstances that have not happened or have already occurred. They stand fundamentally outside the present moment. The only moment that actually exists is the one right now, the one where you are holding this book, maybe a pen in hand, maybe a baby crying in the background, or a semi passing beneath your window, this particular moment where you inhale and the world cries out to you in the form of a crow, or an airplane overhead, or the sound of mail being slotted into the boxes in the hall.

Yoga is not about putting your body into various shapes, though it can be. Nor is yoga about chanting in a room full of others seated in lotus, though it can be. Yoga is, ultimately, a path for realizing that in this particular moment, this one right now, you have everything that you need. You are full. In fullness, there is no room for lack, because, by definition, fullness is already full.

Ancient texts define yoga in any number of ways. The sage Patanjali tells us that yoga is the stilling of the turnings of the mind, while the *Bhagavad Gītā* defines yoga as the ability to remain the same, *samatvam*, no matter what changes around you. In the middle of the first millennium BCE the *Kaṭha Upaniṣad* provides one of the earliest definitions of yoga as "the complete stillness in which one enters the unitive state," while 2,500 years later Sadhguru describes yoga as "the science of being in perfect alignment, in absolute harmony, in complete sync, with existence." What all of these definitions or understandings of yoga have in common, though, is the belief that yoga can only be experienced in the body. It cannot be found in books or prescribed by a doctor or explained by a teacher. Yoga can only be experienced inside each individual. In some ways, the fact that yoga has become a workout in the Western world rather than the path it was always meant to be is not entirely misguided. The body becomes the only source of knowledge in yoga. It is vessel, teacher, and vehicle.

That yoga can only be experienced in the body and that the body is the sole pathway to understanding our connection with every living thing in the universe can feel empowering to those who have an easy relationship with their bodies. If you close your eyes and find familiarity and calm, if you scan your body and experience peace, then the idea that your embodiment is your gateway to freedom probably feels pretty good. However, most human beings do not feel at home in their bodies. In fact, many find the body a source of pain and sadness. We need only look at the numbers of people of all ages, races, and backgrounds who starve their bodies, purge their bodies, cut their bodies, and punish their bodies to see how unsettling our embodiment can be. I think of the writer Roxane Gay, who names her body as both cage and crime scene, or José Orduña, who writes about how his body is made into a weapon by the state, or the terrifying statistics of trans teens who commit suicide because the gender assigned at birth does not align with their experience of gender. Racism, patriarchy, economic inequality, ableism, and homophobia transform bodies into sites of terror and pain rather than sanctuaries. How, then, can we sit with these wounded bodies and let them teach us?

The short answer is that we have no other choice. Each of us has taken birth in this body and in this lifetime. We don't get to choose. And we cannot leave our body any more than we can leave our breath. More to the point, any experience we have in this world is an embodied experience. It happens inside our bodies. The entire world exists within. We can't step outside of ourselves and experience eating or walking or sleeping or crying. We can't see except from our bodies. We can't feel or touch or hear outside of our bodies. We can't think, we can't suffer, and we can't love outside of our bodies. And we can't step into another's body to see what strawberries taste like to them. This is one of the essential paradoxes described in yoga. Sadhguru names it as the human predicament: "the very seat of your experience is within you, but your perception is entirely outward bound."

The knowledge that we cannot share our experience with others nor escape it may sound terrifying or hopeless, but only if you believe that your body is limited to the gross physical body and nothing else. Yoga turns us to the body as the doorway to acceptance, love, and compassion, but it complicates our understanding of what the body is. Historically, the body became central to the practice of yoga between the fifth and tenth century CE, when tantric yogis began to recognize that the body was not just a collection of skin and bones but a vessel for alchemical transformation. Previously, yogis had a conflicted relationship with their bodies where they focused on mastering flesh through mortification and austerities known as *tapas*. The physical body was more hindrance than vehicle. The tantric turn in yoga is what gave rise to Hatha yoga as it is practiced today. By focusing on the body—and in yoga, as we will see, the body is much more than the physical but includes the energetic and spiritual bodies as well as the mind—an individual can transmute the gross into the subtle, not transcending the body but rather moving deeper into the sheaths of the body, to discover that we are, in fact, not simply our physical bodies but rather a life force energy that is found in all living things. We are, a yogi would say, one with everything, and we come to that knowledge by closing our eyes, which challenges the mind's belief that reality exists only in what can be seen. Once we do, we no longer live unhoused.

Yoga and Writing

How does this relate to writing? As a writer, or an artist, or a human being, we must attend to our bodies first before we can move outward into the world, outward with our words, outward with our hearts, outward with our service. We have to take responsibility for our embodiment and deepen our connection to the physical fact of our existence and then, by focusing on the breath and the body, move beyond the physical to connect with the world around us. How can we create characters who are rounded and complex if we have not found compassion for ourselves first? How can we discover the deeper subject of our poetry and our prose if we have not sat with the fear and longing that marks our own existence? How can we attempt to externalize our inner experience—which is the basis of all art—if we are not in touch with the world as it is known inside each of us? It is impossible.

I would argue that you cannot be a writer and not, to some degree, also be a yogi. You may not name yourself a yogi. Others may say you write with wisdom or honesty or clarity, but I would suggest that the writing that speaks most to us is writing that comes from those who are highly aware of their inner experience. In yoga, there is a beautiful name for that inner awareness. It is called *chidākāśa* and derives from the Sanskrit for consciousness and sky. It is the world we see when we close our eyes, the one on the inside of our eyelids. That is our inner sky, and we always want to write from there.

How to Use This Book

The Yogic Writer is meant for anyone who wants to write, and, more specifically, for anyone interested in writing from the sky inside. While the book moves into the body as a source of knowledge and transformation in order to write with clarity and compassion, you do not have to practice postural yoga to benefit from this book. You do not have to be flexible. You do not have to own a yoga mat or know Sanskrit. You simply have to close your eyes and breathe.

Because I follow the yogic path, I believe that everything is connected and that the desire to separate, contain, and, therefore, try to control the world around us brings suffering. *The Yogic Writer* pursues the interconnectedness of breath, body, words, and world by weaving between chapters devoted more to writing practices, chapters focused more on the somatic body, chapters offering breath practices, and chapters, the vast majority, that combine all three. I do not see my breath or the words I am typing at this precise moment to be separate, and I do not think we should be taught that they are. In its structure, *The Yogic Writer* physically demonstrates the union of breath, body, and page.

Furthermore, nothing is exiled on our journey; alchemists inform this book as much as Nobel Laureates. The entire world is our teacher. We just have to open our eyes to that reality, rather than decide only a few offer knowledge. We will explore breathing practices and somatic practices, as well as what makes a scene powerful and a character memorable. I hope you will write a lot. More powerfully, I will invite you to consider who it is that is actually holding the pen. Books exist on yoga practice and books exist on the craft of writing, but these books miss a fundamental truth about our existence: writing does not come from nowhere. It comes from a body marked by its time in the world. *Craft and body are not separate.* The body of your work is your body, whether it takes the form of haiku or novella. Ultimately, this is a book on how to approach writing and life as a yogi would, as someone who is working to remember every day that the rainbow is there, that this moment is full.

Some of you may have been writing for decades, and some of you may just be starting out. Likewise, many of you may be yoga practitioners, while others have never unfurled a mat. I work to include all of you. Charles Baxter, the fiction writer, once said to an audience I was in, "Art is not a sack race." We are always learning to begin again. My goal in writing this book has been to offer a layered approached to yoga and writing so that you can return again and again to the book, always finding something new. I would encourage you to take what you are ready to receive and let the rest go.

Because I believe the breath is where writing begins, the book is divided into four sections that follow the four parts of the breath: inhalation, the pause at the top, exhalation, and the pause at the bottom. In Sanskrit the inhalation is called *pūraka* (again, you do not need to remember the Sanskrit word, just the idea that the breath has a beginning). Not surprisingly, *pūraka* is associated with the season of spring and new starts. This first section, then, attends to the creation of both space and intention, as well as the generation of ideas. The top of the breath, *āntara kumbhaka*, is marked by fullness and summer—physically, it is the moment when the lungs are completely full, denoting abundance and generosity. The second section, then, focuses on the fulsomeness of drafting. We spend time on scenes, and characters, and detail. The exhalation, *recaka*, is experienced in the body as distillation and winnowing. Aligned with the season of fall, this section is dedicated to revision and paring down. We look at chopping limbs and pruning lines. Finally, the winter of the breath, the void at the bottom, no air in or out, is *bāhya kumbhaka*. Such a void appears empty at first but is actually the home to infinite possibility. In writing, the void is the surrender of results and simultaneously a return to what Audre Lorde calls "the nameless and formless, about to be birthed, but already felt."

We are already writers in the same way that the rainbow already arcs over our head. In the Western world, we might be told to open our eyes and see this to be true. Here, we are going to close our eyes instead and turn our gaze to the sky inside. Writing begins not with paper but with the inhalation.

PART ONE

Beginnings—*Pūraka*

1

Writing with the Whole Body

I am a yoga teacher as well as a professor of creative writing. At this point in my life, I find my practice on the mat and my practice on the page are inseparable. Ultimately, they walk the same path, the one dedicated to becoming a better human being. Importantly, becoming a better human has zero to do with whether you can touch your toes, nor does a publication in *Harper's* herald that you have cultivated compassion for yourself or others. The deepest, richest, and most lasting rewards of both yoga and writing have nothing to do with the end point and are concerned entirely with the process. We are always becoming. We never arrive.

At this point, you may not write because you want to become a better person. It has taken me decades to understand that the most sustainable reasons to continue writing are internal and not external. Especially when writers first start out, they harbor dreams of becoming the next Toni Morrison or Ocean Vuong. And they may, in fact, succeed. But that success will not be what sustains them for the long run. No accomplishment carries you. What sustains us in our art is the joy of writing itself, the feeling we have when we are writing, the sense that every so often we find the words that express our inner experience. That clarity—that moment when our inward experience assumes shape in the external world—is called truth. And when we name our truth—whether in fiction, poetry, painting, or dance—we take one step closer to becoming the best possible versions of our selves because truth is always messy, complicated, and hard, and our willingness to name our truth is simultaneously a refusal to let someone else determine it for us.

Too often, in the Western world, we are asked to navigate our day from the neck up. We confuse, I would argue, the mind for who we are. I am Jennifer because I think I am Jennifer. I have been called Jennifer by others. I answer to Jennifer when the barista at Starbucks calls my name. I rarely *feel* my way to Jennifer, rarely ask myself what does it mean "to Jennifer"? We think our way from breakfast to bed, problem solving, negotiating, comparing, contrasting, but rarely stopping to notice how we feel in our bodies or our hearts. In her book *Heart Minded*, Sarah Blondin writes that almost from birth we are asked to leave our hearts and climb into our heads. I always imagine a little ladder when I think about her work. We arrive in this world, she says, as pure light. But within minutes of birth, we experience suffering. A hunger, maybe, or a need for warmth that no one recognizes. We cry, but still the pain remains. She continues, "Pain and sorrow begin to pool inside us, and in our desperation not to feel this pain ... we abandon the one place within us intended to be our safehold." Our heart. We climb out of the heart and into the head where the pain appears lessened by reason and denial.

When my students enter my university classroom, I ask them to bring their entire bodies with them. They may not check their hearts nor their traumas nor their sorrows. If we want to write, then we must be in touch with our whole bodies. To write from the head alone is to write severed. The physical practice of yoga has certainly taught me a lot about being an embodied human being—rather than just a thinking head—but even if you aren't practicing actual poses, you can still benefit from a more Eastern understanding of your body. In yoga, the body is a series of bodies: "sheaths of being" B. K. S. Iyengar calls them. You can think of these sheaths as layers of an onion or a series of nesting dolls. They move from the gross to the subtle; each sheath, then, acting as a bridge, takes us from the manifest world to the place inside us that Iyengar calls "the immeasurable sky within."

In yoga, the outermost sheath, or *kosha*, is called the *annamaya kosha*, or food body. Our physical body is the literal result of what we eat—food becomes flesh. We often only notice our physical body when it is in pain—a bruised shin, a sore elbow. But we can become more aware of the places in our body that aren't calling out. For example, can you, right now, feel your left baby toe? If not, touch your toe and then see if you can keep your consciousness there after sensation subsides. All too often, because of abuse both ordinary and extraordinary, we are made to feel shame about our bodies. We move to the mind to avoid the experience of living in a body that others violate, ridicule, or deem unacceptable. But our physical body is a miracle. It is the way we touch the world and the world touches us. In the breath work we will be doing throughout this book, we will become more aware of our physical bodies as sources of information and experience.

In yoga, the next sheath, or layer, is the energetic body, the *prāṇamaya kosha*, more subtle than the physical body but still felt. To get in touch with your energetic body simply rub your hands together very quickly for thirty seconds or a minute. Then pause and begin to bring your palms away from one another, slowly. Move them together and away without touching them and see if you can begin to feel a kind of heat or force between your palms. If you can't feel it at first, rub your palms together again. You can play with this energy, expanding it larger and larger and shaping it into what in Qigong is called a qi ball—a ball of energy that you create from the energy that runs within and through you. For those of you who need a more scientific explanation of our energetic bodies, we know that on the subatomic level, we are 99.9999999 percent space. Yogis would say that space is energy, and you can become aware of it.

The third body is the mental body, the *manomaya kosha*, or the body made of thought. In yoga, the mind is more complicated than simply cognition. There are different aspects of the mind that include ego and our ability to discern. For our purposes, we can think of the *manomaya kosha* as the running commentary we experience when we are awake and that we temporarily surrender each night when we sleep. If we sit with the mind and the thoughts it generates, we realize very quickly that our mind is wed to the external world, specifically the objects around us. We want some outcomes and don't want others; much of our day is spent sorting through our preferences. These waves of thought can create unease in the body, not to mention suffering. In the next section, when we move to breathing exercises, we will notice how the mind will settle with the breath. The breath slows, the body calms, the mind follows. These bodies, then, are not separate but connected, each bridging to the next. We do not write by head alone.

The fourth sheath in yoga, *vijñānamaya kosha*, is the body that helps us discern the nature of reality. With this sheath, we are arriving at the very subtle. I like to think of this body as the one connected to the heart. An ancient yoga sutra says the heart sees by its own light. In other words, the heart has its own way of knowing, a knowing that is much richer, deeper, and more intuitive than the knowledge created by our heads and based on our senses. Seeing with what the sage Ramakrishna calls the "love eyes" rather than our physical eyes often leads us past the black-and-white thinking that seeks to divide and analyze and instead moves us closer toward connection. We can start to become aware of the *vijñānamaya kosha* by simply taking our attention to our heart space and bringing a loved one to mind. If you have time, maybe try it now. Just sit for a moment, placing your left hand on your heart and covering the left hand with the right, and think of someone who is very dear to you. You might feel your heart begin to swell or even warm a bit. As a writer, you want to know all that your heart eyes have seen.

Finally, the bliss body, *ānandamaya kosha*, is the sheath that allows us, in yoga, to realize our oneness with everything around us. When I talk about this sheath with others, I often have them recall a moment of pure joy, maybe seeing a sunrise, or watching rain fall, seeing the wind made visible by a plastic bag kettling the currents. In moments like these, something deep inside of us, something inchoate, reaches toward, say, the orange cloud or the plastic bag, in wordless recognition. By the time we say, "Look at those clouds!" the moment has passed. The bliss body has nothing to do with whether you believe in god but rather whether you realize the porosity of your edges. When you are in touch with the spiritual body, you see yourself as part of everything—and once you see yourself as connected, you are less willing to harm others, including yourself.

Five bodies in one body, each housed within the next, moving ever more subtle. What a yogic understanding of the body provides is a realization that our body is so much more than flesh or thought. We have to know these bodies exist if we want to write with, and from, them. You can make it a practice to check in with your physical, energetic, mental, emotional, and spiritual bodies throughout the day. Just ask yourself how you feel physically or energetically or emotionally. Give your mental body a color or a texture. Ask which body is making the most noise, which body has gone silent. Knock on the door of the bliss body and see if anyone answers. Hold your own heart. See if you can travel from flesh to energy to consciousness to discernment to joy and then back again. Notice what there is to notice.

2

Born to Write

In fifth grade, my teacher announced that our class would be hosting a carnival as a way to understand the market system. She told us we could sell anything we wanted at the carnival and that she would track how much money each student made. Desks would serve as booths, parent volunteers would help with setup, and we were to "be creative." Even at the age of ten, I remember being unsure of how to spontaneously generate creativity and how, exactly, creativity was connected to the market, but I was determined. We had been learning about bank accounts and loans and how to calculate interest rates for weeks. In my backpack, I carried my mother's checkbook, devoid of checks but with deposit slips remaining. From a distance, my classmates could not tell what I signed as I tore—slowly so that the sound carried across the classroom—each "check" from its binding.

The day my teacher announced the carnival, I went home abuzz with energy. While my friends and I regularly held informal swap meets on my bedroom floor, trading Star Wars cards and Hello Kitty stickers, I knew that, for the market at school, I needed to sell something new, something shiny, something that all of my classmates would value. I chose to sell my poetry.

As you can imagine, it did not go well. I sat inside my desk-booth the entire afternoon of the carnival and sold not a single poem. No one wanted my poem about rulers ("Inch, inch, inch/they pinch every inch on a ruler/for it is a schooler") or my poem about sunsets ("The sun died another day"). Instead, they all bought the rock candy Robert Hunter offered, red prisms of sugar clumped on a stick. The line for his wares ran into the halls.

Toward the end of the day, my teacher took pity on me and came to my booth. She said she wanted to commission a poem from me, one about police officers. My shoulders sank, but I took out my notebook and tried to think of something beautiful to say about a profession I knew nothing about. My page remained blank, my till empty, and I chastised myself for not selling chocolate chip cookies or brownies, something that did not ferry my heart.

So much could be said about that carnival afternoon. I often name it as the first time I experienced rejection for my writing, as well as the first time I understood, unconsciously, that writing had to come from within, not without. It's also the first moment where art and marketplace became wed for me. All these lessons would inform my understanding of myself as a writer—mostly negatively—for decades to come.

I imagine you have had similar experiences. My guess would be that maybe you, too, could trace your understanding of yourself as a writer back to origins marked by shame, rejection, or sadness. Maybe it didn't happen when you were ten. Maybe it was a friend questioning what you planned to do with a degree in English. Or maybe you haven't even admitted to anyone that you want to write. Most of the writers I know tell similar stories. Many of them still refuse to call themselves writers.

From an early age, we are taught to seek external validation for our self-worth. It begins, unintentionally, with our parents, who all too often project their needs and desires onto us. But the story is quickly taken up by a schooling system that is bent on comparison, measurement, and ensuring that children sit on their pockets. There are millions of ways, largely invisible, that we are taught to seek outside affirmation, but the result is that we often allow others to determine if we are good or bad, worthy or worthless, a writer or a fraud. When we look outside ourselves for validation, we give up our own power, from a very young age, to determine not only who we are but how we can best express our unique self. Comparison, the instinct to survive, and the drive to succeed lie deep in our DNA as human beings. And being named "the winner" brings material and cultural benefits. No doubt. But the harm to artists and the creation of art is great. The direct result of tethering our understanding of ourselves as writers to others' acceptance, adoration, and love is a child crying in her bed at night, her poetry journal halted in fifth grade, telling herself that she was stupid to have shared her words.

You are a writer. Already. Right now. There will never be a moment when some glowing figure from the sky taps you on your shoulder and ordains you. No publication, no award, no amount of recognition will ever make you feel like you have arrived. The only person who can confer the role of writer on you is you. And you are a writer because you write. My guess would be that you write a lot, have been writing for a long time, and, most importantly, use writing to navigate your world. Whether you write fiction or nonfiction or poetry, you write to know: to know yourself, to know your characters, to know your past, to know what it is you plan to do, as poet Mary Oliver says, "with your one wild and precious life." Clay does not call you; chemical equations are fine but they do not sing; when the sun pierces leaden clouds to reveal a ladder of light, you don't reach for your paints. Rather, maybe you wonder if ladders can be made of light and if that is the best metaphor to capture the way your heart unfolds at such grace.

A writer is not something we will become one day when the teacher tells us, or a degree is conferred, or we reach the age of forty. A writer is something we realize within ourselves. We peel back the layers of shame, dampen the voices that told us we couldn't, stop listening to the people who connect writing to marketplace, and we allow our inner writer, the one who has been with us almost since the day we first spoke, to step forward. The poet Rainer Maria Rilke implores young writers to "keep growing, silently and earnestly, through your whole development." "You couldn't disturb it any more violently," he continues, "than by looking outside and waiting for outside answers to questions only your innermost feeling, in your quietest hour, can perhaps answer." Do not give away your power to determine how you will spend this one wild and precious life. It's a choice. You can wait for the rest of the world to tell you who you are or you can pick up a pen.

3

Set Your Goats to Roam

Some months ago, I was hiking in southern Utah, just outside Moab, with my parents, husband, and one of my children. We found ourselves alone under the desert sky, surrounded by oceanic emptiness. The desert is a place of elemental beauty that only yields its treasures to those who pay close attention. Unlike, say, the Hoh Rain Forest in the Pacific Northwest, populated by enormous moss-covered trees with immediate bearing and consciousness, the desert is reticent and unshowy. The land in Nevada and southern Utah has long been deemed empty, worthless, and something one must drive through to arrive at the oasis of California. I love the desert for its restraint, its withholding, its secret keeping, and I am honestly happy for everyone else to just keep driving so that I can sit amid red rock, blue sky, and the occasional juniper.

That day we were hiking Hidden Valley trail, a trail that climbs steeply up the side of a mountain and then opens onto a valley. Don't think trees and grasses and sweet little cows chewing dandelions. Like the desert itself, this valley will check your assumptions, point out your preference for the abundant, the verdant, the green. We walked along the valley floor, dotted by boulders and canopied by sky, until finally climbing to a saddle where crimson hoodoos stood sentinel and a raven stroked the air above our heads. Rather than stopping there, a pass where most hikers remain before trekking back down, we continued along a path that humans have been using for thousands of years to arrive at a mesa. The formation rose from the surrounding bedrock to sail the earth like an enormous ship. As we followed the cliff band around the mesa, we came to panels of rock art, petroglyphs, that ancient people carved at a time when woolly mammoths still roamed the land. The figures ranged in color from umber to black to white, and most hovered right at eye level. The paw of a six-toed bear, a careful line of mountain goats descending in size, a spiral that swirled forever inward. Desert air is finer than a library archive for preservation, so the panels are truly some of the most outstanding examples of this ancient art form. Some human figures towered with lightning bolts for arms and horns rather than a helmet or headdress. Some of the figures embraced, a figure inside the belly of another, held. They remained vibrant, sharp, and energized. My impulse (not followed) was to place my hand along the curves another had carved. To touch the past. At a moment in human history when mastodons gathered in herds, humans took time to inscribe what lived within.

Flannery O'Connor is often quoted as saying, "I write because I don't know what I think until I read what I say." At first, that may sound strange—that we have to read what we have written to know how we think about the world—but the mind runs in frenzied currents; it rarely eddies in a single place. Writing, though, stills. It garbs our inner experience in the dress we call language so that we can now see what was unseen, watch how it moves, and learn its preferences, patterns, and limitations. More importantly, each of us lives at the intersection of everything that has happened to us; the experience of being in this body, in this lifetime, living on this planet, is entirely unique. No one else will have ever that same body, sit at the same intersection, clothe their inner world in the same dress. Our individuality is both our gift and our burden. We see the world through singular eyes, but no one will ever understand entirely what it feels like to be us. Unique but alone. Which is one of the main reasons why humans have made art: to articulate their singular experience of this particular birth. Art (and here I mean small "a" art, not capital "A" Art) becomes a kind of table, made by an artist; it is their invitation to others to gather around. The human who carved a line of mountain goats onto a panel of rock in southern Utah 2,000 years ago was probably not thinking of their future audience. They were not making Art. They were not seeking compensation. They were trying to reflect their inner values and experience. The fact that I want to place my hand along the backs of their goats suggests that their impulse to create becomes an invitation to connect. I am grateful for the chair at the table that they offer.

Not all writing, of course, is an effort on the part of an individual to understand what they know to be true. Some writing is transactional (contracts and legal documents), some writing is fundamentally informative (the directions to assemble a humidifier), and some writing is documentary in purpose (a bank statement). But the writing we do as people born to write is a way of knowing and understanding, *our* way of knowing and understanding. We write because we have to. And we wait to see what we know. The writing leads us. The writing fills us. The writing is both means and end. Rilke tells those possessed by writing to "build your whole life in accordance with this necessity; your whole life, even into its humblest and most indifferent hour, must become a sign and witness to this impulse." We need to intentionally build a life of writing, a whole life, one that stands as sign and witness to our daily attempt at transmuting our inner reality into words on the page. Most importantly, we do not need to know anything to begin. The writing reveals what we know to be true. We just attend.

If writing is how you make sense of your world, how you express what thrums deep within you, then there is no halfway. Half knowing is partial and even dangerous. Half a sentence will forever remain unintelligible. Instead, as Rilke writes, you bind yourself to the process that leads to understanding, to knowledge, a process that helps you become a better human being, and you make your mark, whether on rock or page. And you do it because of the joy you feel, fleeting indeed, when what you have placed outside your body faintly resembles what you experience inside. You set your goats to roam, your circle to spiral, the lightning to charge the imagination of another. No one else can do this work. The dancer Martha Graham writes, "There is a vitality, a lifeforce, an energy, a quickening that is translated through you into action, and because there is only one of you in all time, this expression is unique. And if you block it, it will never exist through any other medium and will be lost." No one else can hold your pen, nor would you ever want them to.

4

Breathing to Write

From the moment you were born until the moment you die, you will never be outside your breath. Unlike cells that die every seven years or the skin that is shed, your breath is the single most faithful companion to your days. We breathe some 22,000 times a day, and almost all of those inhalations and exhalations go unnoticed. Even though we cannot step outside the breath, we often fail to notice its presence, a presence more intimate even than the heart because we feel it more readily.

The vast majority of us not only do not pay attention to our breath, we actually limit our breath, content to pant at the top of our lungs. Like a dog, we take short, shallow breaths that keep us alive physically but neglect to realize the full potential of our lungs. Many books on writing will begin with the importance of brainstorming or keeping a writing notebook, but I believe writing begins where our experience on this planet begins: the inhalation.

If you were a student in my university class, you would arrive on the very first day and be asked to close your eyes—before roll, before introductions, even before ensuring you were in the right classroom. In case you have never been asked to close your eyes in a public, institutional space, I will say here that it can be scary. As visual creatures, human beings generally don't like to close their eyes, unless they are safely tucked into their beds. Additionally, universities are generally not places where students are asked to do anything other than listen and take notes. They are rarely asked to make their bodies vulnerable.

But we do it. On the very first day. And we sit in the relative silence of an institutional setting, the nervous shuffle of feet, someone in the hall, a cough, a laugh from another classroom, maybe the low growl of a leaf blower heard through a window left open in the early fall. I wish I could sit with you right now, together, with our eyes closed. The experience of breathing together cannot be replicated on the page. But we are all writers, so we know there is always a gap between experience and words. We get as close as we can. To that end, here and throughout the book, I will offer opportunities to practice an intentional breath. We begin with the most basic practice: a four- and six-count breath.

Breathing Exercise One

Come to a comfortable seat. Close your eyes and rest your hands gently on your legs or your lap or the table in front of you. Pull your spine away from the chair and sit tall but not forcibly erect. Feel yourself a tree, rooted at the base, aspiring to light. Remove the tension in your face, releasing your jaw and the space between your eyebrows. Feel the skin on your cheeks go slack. Let your shoulders rest down and away from your ears. Feel your feet against the ground if in a chair or your legs against the earth if you are seated on the floor.

Breathe here. Don't change your breath; just take your awareness to it. In yoga, the natural breath is called the *ajapā japa*, and ancient yogis saw the sound of the natural inhalation and exhalation as a mantra being chanted by the body from birth. For them, the sound resembled the Sanskrit mantra: *so'ham*. Freely translated: I am that. The natural breath, then, repeats this mantra 22,000 times a day. *So'ham* affirms that what lies deep inside of me—the Self beyond the self—is the same as the Self that resides deep in you. Some might call that a soul. Others, the prick of consciousness. Others, beauty itself. Or truth. Or, for the physicists, light. As you begin, simply bring your awareness to your breath, the gentle inhalation and exhalation, the mantra your body chants all day long, affirming your connection to everything.

As you sit here, know that you breathe with all living things on this planet: any people in the room with you right now, the people in your family of choice, the stranger you passed this morning when out for a run, the rabbit that ran at the approach of your footsteps, the hawk that shrieked an alarm. In addition, your exhalation provides the inhalation for the trees around you. And you, in turn, ingest the exhalation of leaves into your body with each inhalation. There has never been a moment when you stopped breathing. This breath, the one right now, is threaded to every breath you have ever taken. No stitch has been dropped. This breath can be followed directly back to the moment you left the womb.

Breathe.

Now begin to take a more intentional breath. In yoga, regulation of the breath is called *prāṇāyāma*. For now, simply focus on the inhalation. Take the next inhalation deep into your belly and let the belly fill, get round, soft. Then watch the inhalation travel up the body to spread the ribs like birds' wings, then finally arrive at the top of the lungs where it lifts your collarbones. That is a complete inhalation. Take a few breaths just noticing how a full inhalation reaches far beyond the physical organ of the lungs.

Now turn your awareness to the exhalation. At the top of the next inhalation, feel the natural U-turn of the breath and follow the exhalation down the body, watching the air leave the body from the collarbones, down to the chest where the ribs knit together, and then to the very bottom of the lungs, deep in the belly, where the navel pulls into the spine. Practice this yogic three-part breath for a few breath cycles. Inhale: belly, chest, collarbones. Exhale: collarbones, chest, belly. Feel the air irrigate your lungs, filling all the little cracks and crevices that have been neglected all day long because you were content to pant at your collarbones. Don't reach or grab for the breath. It is a gift freely given by the universe. Accept.

Finally, add a breath count to this practice. On your next inhalation, inhale to the slow count of four and then exhale to the longer count of six. Try to take in the same amount of air you inhale at one as you do at four. Same with the exhalation. Steady and even. When we extend the exhalation two counts longer than the inhalation, we are activating the parasympathetic nervous system, the part of our nervous system that calms us. We don't have to do anything other than exhale two counts longer. Feel your body start to settle. Your physical body but also your mental body. This breath is magic. It will save you. Breathe for at least two minutes with a four- and six-count breath. Longer if you'd like. When you are ready, slowly open your eyes. Welcome to your writing practice.

I breathe intentionally at the start of my own day as well as the start of class. I will continue throughout the book to describe what happens when we breathe together as well as offer other breath practices, but here I just want to point to the physical benefits. As we breathe with intention, our body settles. In an age of anxiety where many cannot leave their beds in the morning because the idea of eating breakfast let alone passing organic chemistry or meeting with the boss seems like too much, breathing with intention can allow us to calm our body and reclaim our center. I could cite study after study that scientifically proves the health benefits of intentional breathing—better heart rate variability, lower blood pressure, less cortisol in the system—but I am a yogi and yogis trust what they experience in their bodies, not a study involving hundreds. Breathing with intention is the single most important thing you can do to improve both your writing and your life. At the end of the semester, the students I teach at the university regularly tell me that breathing together is the most important tool they learn in my classes. Not scene building, not diction control, not the wonders of non-linear form. Abi Newhouse, a former student, says, "Breathing before class helped me forget that the world outside demanded my attention, so I was able to give all my energy into learning to notice the things I could write about." Another former student, Alyssa Alexander, adds, "Taking a moment to recognize that my breathing is worth paying attention to helped me reconnect with myself and allowed me to work from a more creative space in class."

We breathe until we die. We can either allow those breaths to pass us by or we can use those inhalations to bring us into the present moment, to bring us into our bodies, to allow us to actually show up to the page. This practice takes five minutes at most. Five minutes that allow you to arrive. If you fail to center yourself before you begin to write, then you write both blind and bound.

Writing cannot happen in any place except the present. And the breath anchors you to this moment, this inhalation and the way it fills your body. I would encourage you to make this breath practice—not journaling or reading or drafting—the start of your writing every day. Breathe to write.

5

Effortless Effort

When I am deep in my writing, I lose all track of time. Ten minutes might pass, ten hours, I have no idea. I become like the pitcher that the poet Kabir imagines, the pitcher filled with water and then submerged in a lake: water inside and water outside, no difference between the two. It's not that I have stepped out of time but rather I have stepped into it. I lose all sense of my edges. I am my words.

Many artists and athletes attest to this kind of sublime immersion where the world drops away and they lose themselves in their work. While yogis and those who meditate have long understood this experience of complete oneness (they would call it the beginning of enlightenment), the psychologist Mihaly Csikszentmihalyi offers a more modern understanding that he calls "flow." Flow happens, Csikszentmihalyi tells us, when we are so involved in an activity that nothing else seems to matter. Our concentration is so intense that there is no room for us to think about anything else. You don't think about dinner, or what your friend said, or how you wish you could lose ten pounds. In fact, you don't think at all. You just are. Ironically, these moments of immersion do not happen when we are sitting on the couch doing nothing. We might be tempted to assume that pure relaxation is what leads to a feeling of bliss, but we would be entirely wrong. While the state of flow is nothing short of the ecstatic, we arrive at this state by what Taoists call effortless effort. We work but without working.

Rock climbers know flow. Their lives depend on deep absorption in placing the next cam. Pianists know flow. Their fingers must move more nimbly than thought alone would allow. And writers know flow when they fall into their story, live with their characters, sit with them at the bottom of a well, moss at their backs. Csikszentmihalyi tells us that flow happens when the task in front of us is intrinsically rewarding, that is, when we are writing for ourselves and not the market or the teacher or the bestseller list. Flow also happens when our writing is challenging but not to the point of producing anxiety—a kind of Goldilocks "just right." Anxiety is the enemy of creativity; its focus on a fearful future eclipses the possibility of showing up to the page. Flow also requires enough skill that we are not bored. In some ways, we induce flow but in other ways flow happens when we release expectation and remember that we write because we are called to write, because we love it.

In a state of flow, your mind has no room to comment. It does not have space to project into the future or worry about the past because it is entirely consumed with the present. Often, the mind doesn't even remind you to eat. This kind of absorption is so complete that it can almost appear to take the place of food; it sustains from within.

I personally don't use the term "flow" very often, mostly because I am not steeped in Csikszentmihalyi's work. Rather, because I practice yoga, I use the language of writing in the present moment. What Csikszentmihalyi describes is no different than being in the present moment—which, again, is the only moment that actually exists. The present moment is eternally unfolding and entirely full. The breathing practice in the previous chapter helps us come to the present moment, to learn to recognize the present. Breathing with intention brings us into our bodies and makes us curious about the shape of each breath, where it reaches, how it moves, the way it slides between the ribs. It is where we begin to find that mysterious flow, but it isn't magic. It's work. The more often we remain in the present with the breath, the more apt we are to remain present in other areas of our lives, like our writing.

While some artists may slide into flow without deliberately setting out to do so, Csikszentmihalyi is clear that flow is a state we can create for ourselves. And he knows this because he has lived it. Csikszentmihalyi was a prisoner of war in the Second World War, and much like the Holocaust survivor and therapist Viktor Frankl, he found himself deeply interested in how some people survived such horrors with the ability to still love, while others became the walking dead. What he discovered is that "a person can make himself happy or miserable, regardless of what is actually happening 'outside,' just by changing the contents of consciousness." Before you reject such an idea as a kind of traditional "bootstraps" mentality, it serves to look closely at what he says. Csikszentmihalyi is not suggesting that you just have to choose to be happy. He is saying you have to find what you love and practice that work as a means on its own and not an end. In *The Radiance Sutras*, Lorin Roche says this about effortlessness: "When you allow your attention to be called to something you love, the flow is natural." In other words, if you have been born to write, then you write. And when you write—commit yourself to your task with your entire being and without need for external validation or reward—you have moments, more and more moments, where you become the pitcher in the lake and time stands still. When we "allow our intention to be called to something we love," we become entirely present to that love.

And the present is all that we have. Our choice is merely whether to dwell here with intention and therefore actually inhabit our lives or instead die without ever having lived. Dramatic but true. The moments in my own writing life (or when I am running or practicing yoga or meditating) when I am so entirely immersed in what I am doing that there is no room left in my body to be anywhere else are the moments when I know that I am truly alive. Fear slides away, anxiety, regret, sadness. If you are entirely with what you love, there is no room for anything else. Such immersion begins, simply but not easily, by taking your awareness to this next breath.

6

Form the Circle and Step Inside

When I was fourteen, my family moved from Hawaii to Virginia. My father, a Navy lawyer, had been stationed at the Pentagon, and we returned to the gray skies of Virginia for the second time in my life. Because I was a teenager and too old to share a room with my younger brothers, I was given a room in the basement. A room of my own. Not only did I have my own room but it was in a house that my parents, rather than the military, owned, which meant I could, for the first time in my life, paint my bedroom walls.

I chose pink cotton candy walls with white trim, a seven-year-old's palette. I had been dreaming of my very own room for about that many years, so it makes sense to me that I would choose princess colors. If I could, I know I would have had a canopy bed as well, white posts with gold-swirled finials. Even though my room was in the basement, when I stepped into its pink embrace, I felt light. It no longer mattered that I had left a class of thirty students for a class of nine hundred. It no longer mattered that my contact lenses had not arrived in time for me to begin high school without glasses. Nor did it matter that I walked to the bus stop on mats of wet leaves, no palm trees in sight. Inside the pink walls, I felt warm, surrounded by pillows I had sewed for my bed and beneath a lampshade I created out of white lace. Sitting at the desk at night, illuminated by my lace-topped lamp, I wrote in my diary about my days. Pure teenage angst. No one liked me. I was ugly. So alien did I feel at times in my family that I was convinced I had been switched at birth. I wrote stories as well, horror mostly, fantasy and sci fi, cramped blue lines in a brown spiral notebook seized from the drawer of my mother's desk. One of my fondest memories of the two years we lived in Virginia remains sitting at my desk, the blank page before me, surrounded by the frosting of childhood.

In her famous essay "A Room of One's Own," Virginia Woolf imagines what Shakespeare's hypothetical sister, Judith, might have been able to produce had she not been bound by the gendered norms of her day. Had she a room of her own and the financial support to follow her gifts, might she not have rivaled her brother with her lines? In Woolf's version, Judith kills herself because she cannot bear another day of mopping and baking rather than doing what she was born to do: write. When Woolf suggests that "a woman must have money and a room of her own if she is to write fiction," she is largely focused on material opportunity—literally, privacy and support. When Woolf wrote her essay a hundred years ago, women were not afforded their own humanity. While much has changed, the heart of Woolf's ideas remains true—that we create best in spaces that are marked as special, made our own.

I believe we should write in sacred spaces. Not churches or monasteries or ashrams, though that might be nice, but rather spaces simply set apart. At the root of the word "sacred" is the understanding that what marks something as holy is its distance from the everyday. The sacred is set apart from the secular or the profane and becomes, then, blessed or special. As Brenda Miller writes in "A Braided Heart," a challah loaf, the Sabbath bread for Jews, is not defined by a specific form or the number of braided strands. Rather, she writes, a challah loaf "must only look different from everyday bread .... it need not be braided; it could be circular or oblong or in the shape of a rhomboid for that matter." To be sacred requires only an intention to mark something as so.

Ritual is often used to demarcate sacred spaces—to set them aside. Witches cast circles before gathering as a coven or performing spellwork. In Catholicism, at the moment in mass when the bread becomes the body of Christ, the acolytes ring bells. To open a yoga practice, teachers and students might chant *om* together. These rituals serve to draw invisible lines around, a certain space or action. Those who are participating understand that, even if they have not physically moved, the space itself has been transformed.

Writers, too, create such spaces in which to work. It need not be an entire room; few of us have such luxury. Instead, I would think about your writing space as more of an altar. It might be your desk, or it might just be a corner of a room or of a table. You want to choose a place that is convenient and one you can claim as your own. Again, the space itself need not be fancy; it is your intention alone that sets it apart. A yoga studio is a room with four walls until twelve people chant a mantra together; then it becomes a cave of the heart. So maybe you claim the end of the kitchen table or maybe a chair in the den. If you tell yourself you need to remodel your study before you can write, you are doomed. Pick an end table, a lap board, a seat by the window. Designate it as your writing space. Tend it. Care for it. Use it for writing alone. It needs to remain set apart.

The writer Terry Tempest Williams visited our campus decades ago, and I remember her telling us that she always kept a glass of water on her writing desk. Not to drink. Rather she kept water nearby so that even when she wasn't writing, when she was, instead, stuck wandering in the fallow fields all writers must wander from time to time, she knew something was still happening. In this case, evaporation. Anne Lamott keeps a one-inch picture frame on her desk to remind herself to write small. Some writers burn candles. Some writers surround themselves with books that act like talismans, channeling beauty. Again, the physical is not where the power lies. Intention is what matters. You need to mark the space as separate so that, when you enter that space, you know the kind of work you must now do.

Each morning, I sit in front of the altar that Michael and I share. No object on the altar has any material value. Rather, each object reminds me of what I have taken as my central calling: to serve. When I sit in front of the altar in the dark winter mornings wrapped in blankets, I immediately settle. From countless mornings of sitting in this space, a deep part of me knows what lighting the candles means, the sharp smell of incense, the figures and stones and beads that crowd the wooden surface. Because I have marked the space as special—even though the altar is literally in the living room—I recognize the work that must be done. I wouldn't pay bills there. I wouldn't eat breakfast there. I have created a space, with intention, that is sacred; I invite you to do the same. Woolf warns us what happens when we are denied or deny ourselves the freedom to create. Look at her own end to see Judith's played out. Rilke tells us to dedicate our *entire* lives to our art. The very least we can do is claim a table, drape its surface, and light a candle to remind us to burn bright and clear in our work. Bread is bread until its challah. We want to cast a circle and then step inside.

7

Don't Wait for Cadaver Gums

The sage Patanjali compiled *The Yoga Sutras* around 400 CE. A series of aphorisms on yoga philosophy, these slender lines provide the foundation of modern postural yoga practice. Many yoga teachers and students are familiar with Patanjali's first few sutras, the most cited one being the definition of yoga as the stilling of the waves of thought. You only need move a little deeper into the first chapter, though, to find what, to me, is one of the real treasures of Patanjali's offering. In sutra 1.14 Patanjali writes that any success in yoga can only come from practicing for a long time, without interruption, and with devotion: *sa tu dīrghakāla-nairantarya-satkārāsevito dṛḍhabhūmiḥ*. The same is true for any art: long obedience in one direction.

Often we want shortcuts. Ignited by stories of brand-new authors with million-dollar book deals or impatient to write a novel when we have never written a short story, we are often focused on the end. And we want it all now. Art doesn't work that way. Sure there are exceptions, but, for the most part, you must dedicate every single one of those 10,000 hours that Malcolm Gladwell describes in *Outliers*, the hours it takes for musicians and artists to become experts. There are no shortcuts. Period. You begin at the beginning. You begin again many, many, many times. And you remain a beginner.

For how long? Your entire life. Why? Because there is nowhere to go. There will never be a moment when you have arrived. The journey is the end. If you want to write, then you write without a destination or a number of years in sight. In medieval times, an individual interested in learning a craft would become an apprentice to a master tradesperson. A medieval blacksmith apprenticed for at least seven years, a goldsmith, ten. I am an apprentice for life, for I always want to be on the edge of learning, always arriving. Maybe because I was raised in the military and understood the reasons for its strict chain of command, I have been willing to pay my dues. It took me twenty years to write my memoir. Twenty years. Those years were full of frustration and sadness for sure, but they were most marked by consistent practice. Never giving up; always showing up.

If the first part of Patanjali's sutra tells us that we must work for a long time, the second part raises the bar even higher; he insists the work must be uninterrupted. That is *daily* practice. We cannot be weekend writers, like weekend warriors at the gym. We can't spend five days a week watching reruns of *Gilmore Girls* and then decide on Saturday to become a writer for a few hours. In the previous chapter I wrote about how ritual can be used to mark our writing space as sacred, but writing requires a second understanding of ritual as well—that it has to be as daily as our breakfast, the news, the dog at the door wanting to go out. In other words, writing needs to become the kind of habit where, when we forget to do it, we feel slightly off center.

For decades, I did not floss my teeth. Brushed them, sure, twice a day. But flossing always felt too hard, or I couldn't find the floss, or it hurt. In my mid-thirties, I learned that my gums were receding, exposing the tissue and bone to permanent damage. The dentist sent me to an oral surgeon who scheduled gum surgery right away. The morning of my surgery, the surgeon gave me two options for replacing the gum tissue that I had lost: they could harvest it from the roof of my mouth, incurring additional incisions, or they could use gum tissue from a cadaver. I chose the latter and woke from surgery with a body no longer entirely my own. While forever grateful that someone donated their living tissue to me, I am also a little wigged out about having cadaver in my mouth. No one can tell. My gums are uniformly pink and healthy. But I know. Of course, I became the most diligent flosser on the planet. I never wanted to spend another day with my head on a pillow, pools of bloody drool gathering beneath my cheek, unable to feel from the neck up. And here's the thing: I have been flossing my teeth every night for fifteen years, and it now feels strange if I have to skip for any reason. A bit naked. Like I forgot to wear underwear when I left the house. The practice became a part of my daily ritual. I would not miss flossing any more than I would leave the house clad only in sky.

You want your writing to feel like that. So deeply a part of your day that it becomes a ritual you never question but just do. It takes time to develop that kind of discipline. Cadaver tissue and the trauma of surgery gave me the motivation to floss regularly, but that is external motivation. The ritual of writing must come from within. No one is ever going to make you write. You have to be the one to commit. Begin small. Ten minutes a day. Low-stakes writing (read the chapter ahead on keeping a writing notebook). You want to experience success here, so make your goals achievable and keep them focused on process (write for a certain amount of time) and not product (a story published in the next six months). I would even encourage you not to set a word count goal. A set time infused by intention is what works best for me.

Finally, Patanjali tells us that a grounded practice requires a third aspect: devotion. Here Patanjali is referring to the kind of devotion that involves giving up all results to sources higher than you: surrender. There is no room for ego in this work—no room for reaching and wanting and craving and grabbing. Instead, we devote ourselves to the work itself. Again, we are returned to the foundational understanding that we must write for ourselves and release our attachment to outcomes. We cannot commit ourselves to years and years, a lifetime even, of daily work if we tie that labor to external reward. No reward will ever be great enough to make that amount of work justifiable on any kind of consumerist scale. We must be devoted, Patanjali says, to the practice if the practice is to ever have a firm foundation.

Sutra 1.14 tells us all we need to know about our calling. If you are born to write, then you aren't casually taking up the robes of a writer like a Halloween costume that you wear once a year. You are committing to an entire way of being in the world. The magic arrives when we realize that our commitment to our practice certainly improves our writing but more importantly clarifies our humanity. In yoga, taken together, this daily practice (a long time, uninterrupted, and with devotion) is called *sādhanā*. At the root of that word is *sat* or truth—not truth as in the opposite of a lie but truth as in realizing what is true about reality: that we are whole, that we are more than our surfaces, and that we shine from within. When we make writing our *sādhanā*, we take daily steps toward that realization on ever-more-firm ground.

8

The Portable Altar

When Michael and I first moved to the West after completing our PhDs, we lived in the small town of Preston, Idaho. Michael had taken a job as a poet at Idaho State University, so he commuted north, while I was teaching at Utah State University and drove the forty-five minutes south most days. We rented a house from a newly divorced woman who took advantage of the fact that we were used to paying the sky-high rents of Ann Arbor and were more than happy to pay $1,000 a month for an entire house. Far too large for the two of us and boasting kitchens both upstairs and down, the house never fit us, but in rural Idaho we didn't have much of a choice.

In the basement, sliding glass doors opened across the valley to the Bear Mountains beyond. The house sat on a flight path for black-faced ibis and sandhill cranes, so our skies were often dotted with lines of birds stretched like beads on a necklace. Michael and I spent a lot of time in the basement, especially in the winter, because it had a gas furnace with a small square window that allowed us to see flames. We called the hulking beige metal box our "fire" and sat in front of its direct heat while the landscape remained locked for months in ice and snow.

My writing ritual began in the dark when I left the house to run. Each morning, I would leave the house in blackness to run those rural roads. In a future chapter, I describe how running is the start of my writing practice, but here I just want to recall leaving the house in blackness to run those rural roads, often threatened by unleashed dogs, almost always accompanied by winds that seemed forever in my face. I ran six miles a day then, so I returned tired and ready for a shower. Within half an hour, I would find myself downstairs in front of the "fire" with a cup of coffee and my journal and laptop. Michael always joined me, and we would write, without speaking, for three hours every morning that we weren't commuting to teach. Three hours was the block of time I had established as necessary for me to "sink into" my writing. Three uninterrupted hours. To others, I would explain that I needed half an hour to journal and then at least two or three hours to actually draft. Met by anything less, like a meeting or a dentist appointment, I would often choose not to write at all. Three hours or nothing. Always facing a landscape that would have made Ansel Adams grab his camera. Bliss.

Then I had kids.

I no longer had three hours. I didn't even have three minutes. Children, especially babies, take your life over. You eventually get a good portion of it back, but not for a decade. I faced two options. I could either never write again—and for someone who sees writing as a way of making meaning out of the world, that was impossible—or learn to write differently. I chose the latter. My altar became portable. My ritual, less ritualistic. I wrote as if I were running an obstacle course, fifteen minutes snatched during naptime, twenty minutes waiting for a piano lesson to be done. You may not have children, but I can guarantee you that you are going to need to learn to move your writing altar. While we, as writers, certainly want to establish a firm foundation of writing every day and writing in the same space, the one we have so carefully imbued with intention, we also have to be reasonable. Unless you are independently wealthy and flocked by paid help, life will intervene. Faced with interruption, surprise, or delay, our first thought will be to give up writing that day, but we have to wait for the second thought, the one that refuses to go to bed without flossing. Then we take out our notebooks (see the next chapter) and write while waiting for Comcast to show up and fix the cable. Or while we stand in line at the DMV to renew our driver license. Or while pumping breast milk. Or while sitting at the bedside of our father who remains weak and unable to rise. Even though we have established our perfect writing space, we cannot wait for it always. We create the habit and then the space can move with us. You can find every excuse not to write. Believe me, I know them all. You want to remove those obstacles and make your practice nimble. At this point, I think I could write in the bathroom of an airplane.

The third time I visited India, I had the opportunity to practice yoga for a month at the Iyengar Memorial Yoga Institute in Pune, India. B. K. S. Iyengar is one of the fathers of modern postural practice and gave us the focus on alignment of the body. Whenever you reach for a prop in a yoga class, you are participating in Iyengar's legacy. The Iyengar Institute is a three-floored building painted white and set amid the flame trees of a (fairly) quiet neighborhood in Pune. We practiced on concrete floors and without air conditioning even though temperatures were in the nineties. In the United States, most yoga studios have floors made of wood or cork and are always air conditioned. Here we tend to privilege physical comfort. But in India, no such luxury exists. You unroll a mat on the concrete and practice.

One day, the teacher told us to keep the mats in their racks; we would, instead, practice on the bare floor. To say it felt strange to no longer have the comfort and familiarity of rubber under my feet would be an understatement. I felt like I was practicing on a different planet. No posture felt the same in my body. My feet slid. My hands grew gritty from dirt. We took *śavāsana*, final relaxation pose, on our backs, our bodies touching one another without mats to keep us separate and isolated. The challenge, of course, was to remain the same in our practice, no matter how the external world had changed. In many ways, I failed, but I will also never forget that particular day or the lesson that I learned. Ritual and routine can found our practice, but change can serve to deepen it.

I miss the quiet time of my early writing life as well as the mountains that rose before me, but I also refuse to be a dainty rose of a writer who needs perfect conditions before they can put words on the page. You only have to be puked on by your two-year-old more than once to come to terms with the fact that art is not a hothouse flower but rather a trench where you either write to save your life or give yourself over to the mud and call it good. Carry your floss with you. Don't be afraid to practice on the floor. You don't fit writing into your life; you fit your life into writing.

9

Casting Language

At the age of twenty-five, I stood at the boarding gate and watched my soon-to-be-ex-husband enter an airplane bound for the mainland and a life without me. I had married young—we had not yet celebrated our fourth anniversary—so it could seem, to an outsider, that this breaking would be somehow mild, like a cold. But suffering does not exist on a continuum for the one who must now sleep in her bed alone. Told by her husband that he no longer loves her, she must grieve the future she will never have; that process is neither short nor easy.

On the way back from the airport that day, I stopped at Ala Moana shopping center and found my way to Honolulu Books. There, on the floor of the store, I spread various writing notebooks at my feet and tried to feel into a future that at that moment I did not want. The return to daily journaling came third in the list of three things I knew might help me in my sadness: running, vitamins, writing. While the months ahead remained unclear—how would I pay rent, should I remain in Hawaii, would my husband return to loving me again—the individual days felt more certain. I could not will my husband to remain with me—I had been begging for six months—but I could keep my body and mind healthy. Decades later, I am struck by the list that I made. These were years long before I practiced yoga, and yet in my three pillars of health and wholeness, I find the care of both body and mind as well as a dedication to daily practice.

I remember well the notebook I chose: a lined, 8.5-by-11-inch, hardback journal with a quilt pattern on the cover. I owned no quilts, did not sew, but clearly wanted generations of women and their daily tasks to guide me in my days. The first line I wrote, once I arrived home to an empty apartment, began, "I am almost 25. A quarter of a century. In some ways I feel old and in others like my life has just begun." I write that line from heart, twenty-seven years after I first set it down. That particular moment of inscription remains for me one of the most powerful acts of writing that I have ever performed. A common enough beginning and a common enough sentiment, but a heroic act nonetheless. I begin with "I"—that slender letter that embodies not only the "I" who wrote in 1995 but also the "I" who is writing here in 2022—and then place myself in time, noting how little I know and yet how much I have already experienced. That was also the moment I became a serious diarist, a habit that has never stopped, and one that has outlasted almost every relationship in my life.

If you are born to write, then you must read and write. You must swim in words, every single day. You probably already do. In a later chapter, I will describe the importance of daily reading but daily writing is where to move after establishing the breath. Just like a ceramicist must throw thousands of pots before they throw the first solid pot, a writer must nail down 10,000 sentences before they write a line that sings.

Keeping a writing notebook differs from drafting a story or poem or an essay. They are two different kinds of writing. Though I am no scientist, my own experience tells me that the two kinds of writing utilize different parts of my brain—the first, more primal, the second, more cerebral. The writing that you produce with an intention to share, no matter how narrowly, is called high-stakes writing. If you are being graded on your work or hoping to publish, the stakes are clearly evident—you will earn an A or a C; your work will be accepted or rejected—but even if you are bringing your writing to just your writing group, the stakes remain high. Others will respond to what you have made. Because the writing that we share becomes writing that is assessed, informally or formally, high-stakes writing causes most people anxiety. When someone tells me they have writer's block, it is usually because they are engaged in high-stakes writing. They are paralyzed by audience.

While we may decide to move to high-stakes writing at some point, we don't want to move there before spending a lot of our time and energy engaged in low-stakes writing. The writing you write in your notebook is low-stakes writing—meant for no one else. If you are like me, no one will ever see what you have committed to the page (my will actually states that my journals are to be burned at my death). In fact, you, yourself, may never return to what you have inscribed. The casting of language alone matters—the process itself—not what you make. A writing notebook is low stakes because the content is immaterial. We think of a notebook as a noun, but it is all verb. You cannot do it wrong unless you just don't do it at all. In fact, I encourage people to be as messy as possible—choose a notebook without lines, a notebook with space to roam, a notebook that can take a beating because it will be used. The writing we set down in our writing notebooks is as close as we can get to invisible ink, writing that is so humble, so grounded, so uninterested in ambition and pretty lines that it only just barely exists as writing as all. Once you turn the page, those words may never see daylight again. To put it another way, your writing notebook represents the first step in externalizing the internal. Like the womb, it needs darkness.

In my experience, the lowest of low-stakes writing can only be done by hand. Computers and typed lines are too orderly and neat to truly abide in the territory of low-stakes writing. Additionally, writing by hand activates parts of our brain, the creative parts, that a keyboard fails to ignite. It does not matter if your teacher told you that your handwriting is illegible—in fact, that's even better. No one ever need read it. A notebook allows you to keep writing as an action rather than solidifying it into a noun, and not just any noun but a precious one, a dainty artifact that requires you to hit "save" before it is lost to time. Write the discarded.

How? Just by writing. I tell students in my classes to write by a timer, twenty minutes at least, and to not censor themselves. Don't cross out. Don't correct. Don't consider word choice. If you need to rant about your roommate's boyfriend or your husband's penchant for midnight snacks, then write that. Make it active and messy, unfiltered and raw. Write until your hand cramps. Complain about how much writing sucks. Be angry at the way your son refused the breakfast that you made him. Let your ugliest self exist on the page—don't exile anything. Just write. Julia Cameron in *The Artist's Way* writes that "all that angry, whiny, petty stuff that you write down … stands between you and your creativity." Getting it down is like clearing your throat. It is a necessary part of the process. Just like you cannot write if you are not in the present moment, you equally cannot write if you are stewing about that speeding ticket you received earlier that morning. Commit the ugly, the messy, the unwanted, the unattractive, the painful, shameful, inglorious parts of your day and your life to the page. Let it be. At some point, you will have cleared space for something more artful and compelling to arrive. Maybe that same day, maybe later that week, maybe a year from now.

What will arrive? I have no idea. I just know that something will show up one day that you will recognize as a sentence, a beginning, maybe what Ann Berthoff calls "ideas to think with." Until that moment, you just keep throwing pot after pot after pot after pot. Fill the first notebook and begin the second; finish a whole shelf of notebooks and buy a new bookshelf from Goodwill. Twenty minutes at least. Every day. *Sādhanā*, daily practice. Try not to miss a day, especially at first. You have to instill the habit (cadaver gums) before the habit becomes your day. In the morning. At night. Whenever you can insist on the space. I like to journal before I begin more high-stakes writing, where I move to a computer and actually carve lines. My own ranting and raving often gives way to the kind of meta writing that helps me figure out what I am actually writing about. In full disclosure, there is a good chance you are going to hate this at first, but there is a better chance that it will become a central part of your life.

Writers write. And we must write lines of dross before we write lines of gold. Your writing notebook contains the dross that you will then alchemize into gold. Remember, there are no shortcuts. No one skips the work. If you don't know what to write, you can read a book like Cameron's *The Artist's Way*, which is full of prompts and inspiration, or work from something like Brian Kiteley's *The 3 a.m. Epiphany*. Me? Well, I ascribe to a sentiment expressed by Flannery O'Connor: "Anybody who has survived [their] childhood has enough information about life to last [them] the rest of [their] days."

10

X Always Marks the Spot

To jumpstart your daily writing, I would like to offer a few writing prompts I find helpful. The first involves crayons and paper, delights we have foolishly ceded to the under-ten. I also like this writing prompt because it appeals to those who think more visually. (An aside here: if you are one who tends toward the visual, you might also draw and sketch inside your writing notebooks.) I learned the general outline of this prompt from a legendary teacher named Tom Romano, whose passion for writing and the teaching of writing remains unmatched, so the process always makes me think of him.

I am not sure what the phrase "writing prompt" conjures for you, but for me it arrives in chains. As the young poet who blanched at being asked to write about police officers, I have long resisted prescriptive forms of writing: write about this. And the word "prompt" itself feels feeble to me, like a crutch, ready to assist. But this is a misguided understanding of how writing prompts work, and the etymology of the word reveals why. While prompt can certainly mean assistance—giving an actor her missed line—its deeper roots are found in the idea of bringing something into the light (from the Latin *promptus*). If I think about a prompt not as a crutch but as a lantern, then the prompt itself becomes less a box and more a path forward. And since we are engaged in bringing the internal into the external, then it makes sense that we carry a few lanterns with us—hence writing prompts.

Scads of writing prompts can be found online and entire books are dedicated to them. In my experience, some writers love writing prompts and fill their notebooks full of them and others avoid them entirely. I would encourage you to hew the middle path. Writing prompts have a place in the process, especially early on when you are casting language. They help generate material, specifically unexpected material, and can take you places you would not travel on your own. An overreliance on writing prompts, however, may indicate a fear of facing the blank page. In those instances, prompts become crutches rather than lanterns because you never have the opportunity to recklessly write about whatever arises. You want a mix.

Lastly, be intentional in choosing your writing prompts. You will have an emotional response to the prompt itself—as in "I like that one" or "I don't like that one." Pay attention to that response. Choose writing prompts that call to you, but also choose the ones you resist. Make yourself write in response to a prompt that seems shallow or difficult or boring or hard. Nine times out of ten, the writing you produce in response to dread will be the writing with the wings to soar.

For this prompt you will need a large sheet of drawing paper and a host of crayons (broken are just fine). If you only have copy paper and a few dried-up markers, then so be it. If possible, you want a large space and lots of colors, also forty-five minutes of time. Begin with the paper and crayons. Now: draw your childhood neighborhood. Don't think. Just draw. I am purposefully giving you no further direction at this point. Just draw. If you had several neighborhoods as a child, pick one. Draw. Use lots of colors. Take your time. At least fifteen minutes.

When you are done, take a look at your drawing. Notice the neighborhood that you chose, if you had options. Consider why you chose the one that you did. Notice the perspective—how close up or far away. How many other houses did you include? How many other apartments or buildings? What were the boundaries of your "neighborhood"—at least for this exercise? Why might that be so? Are those the boundaries of memory or are they the boundaries of how far your mother allowed you to wander? Maybe they are boundaries set by a church or by topography or by the train or by the route you took every year to trick-or-treat. Notice, too, what you did *not* include. Whose houses or apartments were left out and why? What details did you forgo and why would you have chosen to keep them unmarked? Are the undrawn houses the ones without children your age? Or are the absences pointing to religious or cultural differences that you intuited as a child but only now can name? Your drawing captures more than the layout of the streets and the size of the apartment building. Your drawing reveals values and beliefs; it reveals insider and outsider status and whether you felt a part or excluded. Your map begins to point at some of the more complex, and possibly unsaid, issues that circulated in and around your childhood. What you have drawn with your crayons is not neutral but charged. You want to learn to read for the subject under the story.

Now, take a crayon and mark five places on your map that remain an "indelible moment." Romano calls an indelible moment a moment from the past that does not lose its grip. It remains with us, hard and shiny and as vibrant as the moment we lived it. Look at your map and just mark five places where you tie a particular experience to a particular location and the memory vibrates with emotion even if it occurred long ago. Trust the X's that you have placed. They mark buried treasure.

Choose one of these moments and write about it for at least twenty minutes. All five are pure gold, I promise, so it doesn't matter which one you select. You can move toward the one you most want to write about or the one your entirely resist (often the more interesting choice). Write for twenty minutes about what happened long ago on that X. Watch who enters the memory as well as who remains absent. Recall the physical and sensory details. The question when working with memory is always *why* do you remember it this way, so don't worry about whether it is "right" or "wrong." You can choose another X another day. You can also spend time writing about what your map tells you about your assumptions and beliefs. Revisit your map. Regardless of what genre you write, an exercise like this can take you back to the moments that have shaped the person you have become. As writers, we must trust that what we remember, what we carry with us from the past, informs, directly or indirectly, every word that we put down.

11

Picture This

For this next writing prompt (again think lantern not crutch) you need a photo. You can choose any photo, but I would encourage you to find a physical photo. It could even be framed. It's nice to be able to note the materiality of the object as well as the image itself. You can, of course, select one from your phone. You may also choose an image from a magazine or a book. Years ago, I found an enormous, 6-inch-thick, hardcover book of black-and-white photos from the twentieth century at a used bookstore for a dollar. Over the years, I have removed pages from the book and handed them randomly to students in my classes. I have also wandered antique stores collecting photos of people I have never met but that call to me for whatever reason. You need not know the history behind the image. Just choose an image.

Now look at it. This is actually harder to do than you would think. We need to be taught to look. We can glimpse easily, gather the gist, summarize, but deep looking, like deep listening, requires time and patience. It also requires devotion. In yoga, there is a practice called *trāṭaka*, which teaches one how to attend. Traditionally, one who practices *trāṭaka* begins with the flame of a single candle. You light the candle in a dark room and place it about 12 inches away from you at eye level. The practice is only to look, but you must look with your whole being. You also try not to blink, as blinking is thought to disrupt the mind and cause waves.

You might try the practice. Begin with your candle and then remain with your candle, looking at it without blinking, preferably in a darkened room. First, notice the gross object itself. Notice the way the flame dances even without a wind. Notice how the blue center rises and falls like swell of the sea. Allow that sway into your body. Listen to the wax melt, the wick sizzle. Smell warmth. Remain there for fifteen minutes, noticing everything you can about the actual candle. If your eyes water, then please blink. No need to be uncomfortable. Now begin to notice the space around the candle, darkness carved by light. Pay attention to how the darkness gets shaped, how it, too, undulates and shifts. Attend to the relationship between flame and space. Notice the lack of boundaries. When you are ready, close your eyes. See if you can replicate the flame on the inside of your eyelids, the *chidākāsha*, the sky inside. If you cannot, open your eyes again and look longer. Stay there. Watch the flame become a living, breathing being. Let its character unfold. Then close your eyes again.

Once you can reproduce the image in the *chidākāsha*, you know you are close to seeing it. You can bring it inside yourself. For the final aspect of *trāṭaka*, open your eyes again. See the candle before you as a gross object and see only the candle, so that nothing but the candle exists inside you or outside you. Just as you did with the flame and darkness, see if you can blur the edges between your body and the candle. Remember, the flame has already been inside of you. The candle no longer appears behind closed eyes, but your body itself becomes the candle—no space between the one who looks or the object upon which the one gazes just as there is no space between flame and dark. It's almost as if you fall into the flame. As the poet Lorin Roche writes in *The Radiance Sutras* of *trataka*, "With a steady gaze, melt into / The field of space embracing that form." The act of looking, really looking, allows you to close the distance between self and other. Your body candles. Deep looking initiates compassion.

Can we always look at everything with this much longing and intensity? No. But as writers and artists we need to know how to look—how to begin with the gross and then dissolve into the more subtle. This writing prompt gives us this opportunity to practice. Look at your image as if it were a candle. Such a comparison is actually not that far-flung for photos are light writing. They document the signature of the sun, the earth's candle. Look long enough that the image becomes animated, begins to have being and bearing and movement. Notice the edges, and then notice the space created by the edges. You can begin by asking yourself questions related to the gross form—who might have held the camera? How close or far away did they stand and why? What is framed by the photo, and, more importantly, what has been left out? Who isn't in the picture? How might that matter? Why might the picture have been taken? What might have been the intention? How are preliminary readings undone by longer looking? What remains in the shadow?

Then allow yourself to melt into the image, become the mountains or the horse or the daughter or the stranger. No distance between the two. The picture becomes a mirror and you gaze upon yourself. When you are ready, write. Write about the experience of looking, write about what you saw, or write your way into that mirror, into the shadows, outside the frame.

12

I'll Never

I teach several different styles of yoga, everything from restorative to strength. Like the courses I offer in creative writing, variety appeals to me, and I enjoy pushing on the boundaries of one form or style long enough to see it melt into another. At the end of the day, writing is writing and yoga is yoga; we, as humans, just like to reinvent and rebrand because the new and the different sells. That said, one of my favorite styles of yoga to teach is called yin, a practice that is relatively new to the yoga canon but one that contains poses and philosophies dating back thousands of years. In yin yoga, or at least in my yin yoga classes, we never stand up. A cold practice, the poses target the joints and the fascia rather than the muscles. Each seated pose is held anywhere from three to twenty minutes; time flows and you remain.

In yin, a student is taught to come into a pose, say a seated forward fold, and then to find a depth that feels sustainable—sustainable for the length of time you hold the pose and sustainable for a lifetime of practice. Yinsters learn to find a sensation that hovers around three or four on a scale of ten, and they know the sensation they want: dull, bitter, and achy, not something bright and hard. Once they come into the pose and find that sensation—maybe in a forward fold the sensation arises in the lower back or the hamstrings—a yinster resolves to remain still and hold for time. You might try that right now. Just take a simple seated forward fold, with your legs straight and the top half of the body folding over the bottom half. You could consider placing a rolled towel under your knees for support or bending your knees if your hamstrings are tight. Come forward only to the point where you reach a sensation in your body—dull, achy, and bitter—around a three, four, or five on a scale of ten. The sensation will most likely arise in the backs of your legs. Then, and here is the key, you just remain. You take your breath and your awareness to the area of sensation, the target area, and marinate there. Look for places in your body where you are engaging muscles to pull you out of the pose. Our muscles try and save us from suffering. Scan strange places like your forehead or the front of your throat. See if you are engaging muscles there. Notice first how the body resists discomfort physically, how your body is attuned to escape. Here you want to soak in a physical experience that is non-neutral, maybe even uncomfortable, but not painful. Try and stay in your forward fold for a full five minutes in stillness.

Anyone who practices yin will tell you that a yin class is a hundred times harder than a core power class. Moving is rarely the problem for our busy monkey minds. Sitting in stillness—more to the point here—sitting in discomfort, well, we don't really like that. We resist. We think about what we might make for dinner; we repaint our bathroom in our heads; we gnaw on the offhand remark our friend made about our new coat. Yin teaches us to move *toward* the discomfort, embrace it with our breath and awareness, wallow in its eddies. Ultimately, yin shows us how to live with the very real suffering that comes our way in life. And contrary to what you might think, we actually want to walk toward that pain and sadness, what Sri Ramakrishna calls the poison tree, rather than away. The only way out, after all, is through.

Writing, like yin, involves embracing the painful and the difficult. The writing prompt I offer next pushes you into those scary spaces, and it's important to understand, before we even begin, a fundamental truth about pain: it exists. You only have two choices when faced with any kind of difficulty or suffering—accept it or run away. And because pain is part of being human, running away seems a fairly fruitless choice. We can't run away from being human. That's how denial festers and swells—we are trying to outrun our own bodies. Both writing and yoga teach us how to hold the difficult, carry it, and eventually see it fade away, but only when we resolve to remain still and not run.

As you begin this writing prompt, remember that we are engaged in low-stakes writing. No one will ever see what you write here. Ever. In fact, you can burn the pages as soon as you write them because it is only the casting that matters. The prompt itself is simple: make a list of ten things that you would never, ever write about. Number your page one to ten and write down each one as it arises in all its thorny glory. It works best if the list comes from your own life—for example, your own addiction to porn rather than porn in general. Ten things. Don't filter, censor, or hesitate. Ten ugly, scary, shameful, painful things you would never, ever put into words. You can even use code words or symbols. Just get them down.

Then, and you know where we are headed, choose one and write about it. Again, the one you resist the most is the one you probably need to cast. No one will ever see these pages. Keep telling yourself that. Not your mother, your father, your boyfriend, or your son. Write it all down. Write hot and fast. Don't pause. Don't amend. Don't abbreviate or censor. Take at least twenty minutes, twenty minutes where you don't analyze or apologize or hold back. Write.

After this exercise, you may decide that you will never write about this painful moment in any kind of high-stakes venue—even under the veil of fiction or through a speaker in a poem. You may, indeed, burn it all. But notice what it feels like to curve your hand physically around your shame or suffering. Notice what happens when the darkest of darks becomes outlined with letters. Notice how writing begins to give you some control over an experience that before this writing exercise you never wanted to think about again. You are in charge of the version you tell here, and that gives you power over the past.

In yin, we realize that if we take our awareness to discomfort, it dissolves. If, in your forward bend, you try and locate the exact place of sensation in your body, just exactly where in the hamstrings does bitterness dwell, chances are you can't find the exact spot. When you do, the sensation lessens in the light of your consciousness. Or it shifts. Or it changes. Becomes more porous, less dense, more airy. Writing about difficult things works in the same way. Simply fixing what is amorphous, monstrous, and heavy into lines that, no matter what the content, gather in organized syntax on the page transforms the indescribable into the domesticated. We have something now to hold—it no longer has us.

One more word of wisdom about this practice of writing into dark spaces. In yin, when we come into the pose at a sustainable depth, we are looking for what Bernie Clark calls the "Goldilocks position." When we stress our joints and fascia, the stress makes the joint stronger as long as you don't move too far on the scale of sensation. Clark argues that too often we don't stress our joints enough and create what he calls fragility. Too much protection and the joints become sheltered and weak. However, too much stress and the joint will give. In yin, we want just enough discomfort to become stronger, but not so much as to create injury. Goldilocks and the just right porridge.

The same is true for writing into dark spaces. We know that trauma, in particular, can be re-triggered and that sometimes a person isn't in a safe and healthy enough place physically and/or mentally to add any amount of stress, no matter how healthy the stress may appear. I cannot tell you whether you are ready to write into difficult things. I know that such writing can empower and heal and lead to compelling high-stakes work, but I have also seen writers become more depressed and more anxious when they are writing about something that re-triggers trauma. You are the one in charge of your own boat. Typically, my experience has been that as long as the writing remains contained in a notebook—cast but not made public—it heals. I would encourage you to write about the things that keep you up at night, to write about the things that make you feel queasy, even a bit sick. But you need to be ever aware of how your work is affecting you. Writing should fill your well, not deplete. I would hope for you to be brave but ever aware.

13

Inhale the Stars

Take a moment here to check in with your *sādhanā*, your daily practice. At this point, you have hopefully created a sacred space in which to write. That space is marked by talismans and objects that inspire you and make you feel safe and happy. Maybe you burn a certain candle when you sit down to write. Maybe you play a certain kind of music. Maybe you fill a bird feeder outside your window in preparation for your own gathering of seeds. I hope that you have made a space that feels holy to you, set aside, a space of your own. And I hope you are entering that space every day, potentially at the same time of the day, so that, as with flossing, your day feels incomplete if you don't write. When you sit down, the first thing you do is find your breath. You begin with a three-part yogic breath and move to a four-count inhalation followed by a six-count exhalation. You keep your eyes closed, letting your mental and physical bodies soften and settle. Maybe this breath has started to feel like home, so that when you return to it each day the familiar greets you. Then, ideally, you open your eyes and write in your writing notebook for twenty minutes.

Or perhaps you haven't found the stride of daily practice yet. If you haven't yet cemented your *sādhanā*, here is a moment to do so. If you have lapsed, then re-commit. Just like every inhalation is a new beginning, every day offers us the chance to start again. Our life's work consists of trying to become a better human being time and time again. We will never arrive. We are always just starting. Don't chastise yourself; rather inhale and start over. As I write in the introduction, the inhalation contains the power of creation. It fosters new beginnings.

Once again, close your eyes and find the natural breath; just allow the inhalations and exhalations to arrive without any constraint or control. Often, when we take any awareness at all to the breath, our inhalations and exhalations lengthen and soften. If the natural breath deepens on its own, just notice that. After a few rounds of natural breath, move to a yogic three-part breath where you fill all the nooks and crannies of your lungs. Breathe into the belly, then the chest, then the collarbones. Let the breath be effortless, the body floating up on every in-breath and settling down on every out-breath. Once you feel that your lungs are saturated, then engage a four- and six-count breath to activate the parasympathetic nervous system and settle. Breathe this way for a few breath cycles. You are home. Welcome.

Now, turn your awareness to the inhalation. Notice that you never have to ask the universe for the inhalation. You don't have to reach and grab for anything. Honestly, you simply open yourself to receive the inhalation and the air just pours into you. Inhalation is a gift freely given. We entered the world, every single one of us, on the inhalation. Breath was the first gift we were offered at birth. And, so far, the inhalation has never left us.

In the four parts of the breath (inhalation, pause at the top, exhalation, pause at the bottom), the inhalation is both spring and creation. *Prāṇa*—both the gross breath and the more subtle aspect of *prāṇa*, which is lifeforce energy—keeps us alive. As fragile human beings, we need food, water, breath, and shelter. Without any one of these, we die. Each inhalation, then, creates the possibility of continuance. Because we inhale, we remain. Inhalation moves up and out when we breathe. See if you can feel that energetic movement of the breath. It begins in the belly and then both rises and moves outward, so that our collarbones actually move away from one another at the top of the inhalation. That movement, in yoga, is a *pranic* movement (as opposed to down and in, which is *apanic*). That the inhalation moves up and out makes sense because inhalation allows the body to grow. The oxygen coming into the body with the in-breath replenishes our blood cells, feeds the heart, and nourishes the brain. Try and be in touch with this blossoming of breath as you sit. Watch it swell in your body. If you stay with the inhalation long enough, you begin to realize you are inhaling far beyond the physical perimeter of the lungs. Maybe the inhalation begins in the toes and fountains at the crown of the head. The feeling, once you are attuned to it, is nothing short of euphoric. Every in-breath lifts you up toward the sky. Every in-breath reminds you to open up and out. Every in-breath eventually arrives at fullness, completion, wholeness.

The inhalation teaches us gratitude for all that is offered. If you are feeling down or depressed, dark and low energy, then focus solely on your inhalation. The entire universe is drawing you up toward the light and the sky. Not only that, but every inhalation, on the level of the particle, contains the breath of every human being who has ever lived on this planet, as well as the exhalation of the trees and the stars. You are being filled by constellations when you breathe in. All the great writers and artists from the past commingle in your lungs. Let yourself open to the joy of the inhalation. It is reminding you that creation cannot be purchased, willed, forced, or even sought. Rather, creation arrives merely by opening yourself to it. It pours into your body.

14

Fiction Doesn't Exist

As a child, I could never remember whether fiction or nonfiction contained fact. The label of nonfiction baffled me. After all, negation typically undoes the noun it negates—a non-sequitur, for example, has no sequencing—so nonfiction always seemed like the not true. Wrong. I was well into high school before I could keep the terms straight and remember that I liked fiction. For the record, as a child growing up in the late 1970s, I also could never remember if I was supposed to like disco or rock. All too often, I turned toward either Robert Hunter or Steven Slater, the two "bad" kids that I, as a "good" kid, buffered in middle school, and asked them which one I liked. Rock, they would tell me, and I would try to remember that, even though my spiral notebook had an image of the Bee Gees running through the surf.

In the past thirty years, decades in which creative nonfiction has claimed its status as the fourth genre (along with fiction, poetry, and drama) and has even threatened to displace the sale of fiction at the cash registers, calls have repeatedly been made to change the name of nonfiction to something more poetic or more accurate or just less negative. Literary nonfiction has been suggested or literary journalism, or narrative nonfiction, or just simply essays, or research-based creative writing, the list goes on. For the most part, the term "nonfiction" has remained even as we understand how it fails.

The writing prompts I have offered so far all seem to prepare creative nonfiction writers, memoirists in particular, a place to begin. But I want to suggest that all art, specifically all literary art, is rooted in our past experiences as human beings—even if we set a story on Mars. Further, I would argue that writers of any genre must begin their work by sitting with their own humanity—coming to terms with the fact that all of us, at the deepest level, are trying to do our best even though we repeatedly fail, repeatedly harm, repeatedly hurt the ones we love the most. For me, all writing begins with compassion for ourselves that we then extend to our characters and speakers, even if they have ten eyes or strangle baby chicks for fun.

In 1978, John Gardner published a book titled *On Moral Fiction*. While many today would call his ideas outdated, old-fashioned, and overly idealistic, his basic premise cannot be wholly dismissed when considering why we write or paint or dance or sing. In general, Gardner makes a case for honoring and valuing fiction that is moral—by which he means, on one level, not commercially driven and, on another, concerned with inspiring readers toward a kind of universal truth. In a famous passage, he writes:

> True art, by specific technical means now commonly forgotten, clarifies life, establishes models of human action, casts nets toward the future, carefully judges our right and wrong directions, celebrates and mourns. It does not rant. It does not sneer or giggle in the face of death, it invents prayers and weapons. It designs visions worth trying to make fact. It does not whimper or cower or throw up its hands and bat its lashes. It does not make hope contingent on acceptance of some religious theory. It strikes like lightning, or is lightning; whichever.

Modern writers and critics rightfully recoil at the idea that art is not allowed to rant, that it cannot sneer in the face of death. We live in an age where art more often disrupts and perhaps even disgusts than celebrates, and we are far beyond a belief in the existence of "right and wrong directions." But Gardner's central contention—that fiction has a duty to affirm universal human values—remains key *not* for its emphasis on universality but rather for its emphasis on the connection between making art and being human. Art is made by individuals who eat, sleep, laugh, cry, and poop. Art comes out of our humanity, our experience of being a human being, out of what it means to wake up as a three-year-old in your warm bed while your mother hums in the kitchen and sunlight spills across your bedspread; what it means to send your child to school when you worry they are being bullied and have to watch them climb the stairs into the maw of a bus that will take them away from you; what it means to lose the bottom part of your leg to cancer and have to make choices at the gym about when to remove the prosthetic and when to tough it out; what it means to step outside in the summer and smell the pine trees as they warm in the day; what it means to want a pregnancy that you will never have, a job you will never have, a partner you will never have, a body you will never have; what it means to taste childhood in orange sherbet. Art cannot come from anywhere else except inside of us. We make art. In that way, all art, including all fiction, begins in the true and the real. It has to. And it begins with understanding our own experience of being human even if the characters we will animate are not.

In *The Atlantic*, fiction writer Mary Gordon offers an update to Gardner's call for a kind of art that "establishes models of human action." Importantly, she doesn't reject Gardner, doesn't try to argue that fiction has no obligation to explore the human predicament. Instead, she seeks moral complexity. She writes that fiction is

> uniquely qualified to provide some virtues: the virtues of compassion, openness, and attentiveness. Serious fiction is uniquely qualified to combat the sound bite. It says to us that the truth of human beings is often more complicated than we think. What we might like to call the truth is often made up of several truths, including the first thing we thought, its opposite, and something in between.

Gordon, like Gardner, points to the work of fiction to reveal what it means to be human, but she takes pains to suggest that those truths are neither singular nor static. For Gordon, truth remains at the bedrock of fiction, even if that truth is contrary, fraught, and messy. I think it is worth noting that the first virtue of fiction that Gordon lists is compassion. At its root, compassion means to suffer with. Etymologically, that passion was historically connected with the suffering of Christ on the cross, often seen as an ultimate kind of suffering. In Sanskrit, the word *anukampā*, compassion, means literally to tremble beside. To be compassionate is to tremble with another—and the very first Other that we must suffer with, sit with, and embrace is the version of ourselves that we have trouble accepting.

Whether you are a poet, a fiction writer, or a memoirist, I would argue that your early writing should be focused on excavating your past and finding compassion not just for your own shortcomings and failures but also for those who struggle alongside you—your parents, your partners, your coworkers, and your children. We must begin with ourselves because we are the only human beings that we will ever really know. You may be in love with many, but you will only know intimately one human being: you. And then from that examination, excavation, exploration of your own humanity—learning to love yourself despite your mistakes and failings—then, and only then, can you create characters, personae, speakers, and narrators who readers will follow, love, despise, and sorrow for. Art is moral because it illuminates our limits and then embraces them. As a writer, you must honor and embrace those limits in yourself before you create them in others.

15

On Fire

When I began taking yoga classes more than twenty years ago, no yoga studios existed in Logan, Utah. In fact, the classes I took in the early 2000s were held in the middle school gym. We rolled out our mats beneath the basketball hoops and remained in our sweatshirts to stave off the cold. Decades later, I can take my pick of places to practice—and not just at yoga studios. Rec centers, rock gyms, hospitals, and community centers offer yoga classes here in town. My two children, both in high school, can choose a yoga course for PE and will take those classes in a room filled with mats and props. The university where I teach offers a minor in yoga studies. Yoga is everywhere. And that is wonderful. But I am also constantly struck by how science, education, and medicine have somewhat recently come to realize how important yoga and mindfulness are for our well-being. Discoveries appear in the news all the time about how meditation improves, say, the heart rate or a student's ability to score well on a test or a violinist's performance in a concert. Yoga, as a practice and philosophy, has been around for at least 3,000 years, and likely much longer. And in those eons, yogis, many of whom had to take to the forests or the outskirts of town to practice, have attested time and again to how meditation, breath work, and *āsana* calm their minds, extend their lives, and take them to the ultimate truth. As I wrote earlier, Westerners tend to distrust bodily experience and put too much faith in numbers. Part of me just shakes my head when I read yet another study that "proves" that when you pay attention to your breath your cortisol output lessens. We trust a graph but less our own experience of embodiment.

I think, though, if we are honest, we would recognize that the promises of yoga to help us become better human beings is actually a truth that we, as Westerners, already know but have forgotten. Our language reminds us. When we say that we have fallen head over heels for someone, or that an insult really burns us up, or that our heart overflows, or that we are up to our necks in stress, we are using metaphors to underscore the fact that joy, sorrow, trauma, ecstasy, and love reside in the body, in the tissues of our body. We are affirming in our language the mind-body connection even if we disregard it at a more conscious level. The body knows.

As George Lakoff and Mark Johnson describe in their book *Metaphors We Live By*, a metaphor reveals our deepest values and beliefs. A metaphor makes us naked, reveals what exists below our conscious thinking. If we marshal evidence in our essay, then we see writing as war. If we believe time is money, then we work late and miss our daughter's childhood. If we say the US government bombed Hanoi, then we don't see ourselves individually complicit. In these examples, a truth gets revealed that we, as the ones casting language, may not even fully know.

In fact, knowing itself can be complicated if we pay attention to the language we use to describe *how* we know. Often, for example, we say that we feel something in our gut or that we are trusting our gut. We name the belly as a source of knowledge. The vagus nerve is a network of fibers that runs from the brain directly to the internal organs and from the internal organs directly to the brain. This supercharged highway, the thoroughfare of the gut-brain axis, is both a physical road and a biochemical path. Named "vagus" because it wanders—affecting many parts of the body—the vagus nerve is *the* primary nerve of the parasympathetic nervous system, the part of the body that either calms us down when activated or allows us to spiral when shut down. Because the vagus nerve functions outside the control of the central nervous system, some scientists call it the "second brain." Others, like Resmaa Menakem, call it our "soul nerve." Our gut, it turns out, knows as much and possibly even more than our prefrontal cortex, the part of our brain that allows for higher thought and separates us from other animals. In short, it is not happenstance that we experience loss as a punch to the gut or commit to action based on a feeling in our gut or agree to a second date because of the butterflies in our stomach. Those are not just metaphors. They point to the direct connection between belly and brain and reinforce the vast experiential knowledge of human beings over time who understood that insight, courage, despair, and trauma are located in the physical body. Science has caught up, but language reveals that we have long known about the body-mind connection.

Which is a very roundabout way of saying that I believe we must learn to write from our second brain rather than our first. The head is the territory of the prefrontal cortex and the frontal lobe—the parts of the brain engaged in categorizing and judging and negating and problem-solving. The prefrontal cortex allows us to make decisions, weigh options, determine our future, while the frontal lobe completes our Calculus problems. In writing, we don't want to invite that brain to the party—at least not early on. We want to pay attention to the second brain, the one that resides in our belly, in a space far below parsing and ordering and naming and distilling—the one that wanders the body, touching our entirety.

It's hard to get there. Really hard. Our frontal lobe and prefrontal cortex are so good at their jobs. We have to trick ourselves back to the gut, especially at first. What follows is a writing exercise to help you return to your belly. You will need to write as you read the rest of this chapter for it to work. Don't read to the end. So stop here and grab your notebook.

Write for ten minutes about your first experience with fire. That's all I will offer. Write about your first experience with fire. Don't continue until you have done that.

Now, stop. Pick up your pen. Breathe.

Open your eyes and write for ten minutes about your most recent experience with fire. Just write.

Don't read any further until you have done that.

Don't read any further.

Don't read any further.

Don't read any further.

Don't read any further.

Stop. Pick up your pen. Close your eyes. Breathe.

Open your eyes, and write for ten minutes about a third thing. Don't question. Don't sort. Don't consider. First thing that comes to your mind when I ask you to write about a third thing. Follow that.

You can do this writing exercise with any of the elements or really with any subject. You just want to give yourself time to sink into a subject so that you are following it narratively—the story about fire—and then you want to move from your gut to see what arises that has everything and nothing to do with fire. No matter how random the third thing is, it is related to fire. Your job, as a writer, would be to figure out how.

Warning. If you are spend time thinking your way to the best third thing, you are sunk. To write from your gut requires that you unlatch yourself from the part of your mind that likes order and symmetry. Trust your gut. We, as humans, have been doing it far longer than making bricks, forging steel, or amassing large-scale data sets that prove the connection between body and mind. Your body knows.

16

Archives Aren't for the Dead

The same summer that I was divorced, my great-aunt handed me the diary of my great-great-great-aunt Annie Ray, a woman who homesteaded in the Dakotas in the late nineteenth century. Actually, what she handed me was a stack of typed pages, her transcription of Annie's diary, complete with Liquid Paper corrections. I began to read the diary on the first night I went out for dinner alone. An act of courage, it seemed at the time, to sit at a bar and drink a glass of wine by myself while the restaurant around me exploded in laughter and happiness. If I were honest, I would say that I took those transcribed pages with me that night as a kind of shield, something to do while I sat there, alone. These were the days before cell phones. Instead of Instagram, I scrolled through the winter of 1881 and the summer of 1882, trying to understand what it meant to be a woman almost exactly my age, living in a claim shanty alone while her husband headed to the silver mines in Colorado to shoe horses.

Annie, though, would not tell me the story I wanted to hear. Instead, in her very short entries, she wrote about baking bread and mopping, darning socks. It would take me a few years in graduate school studying women's autobiography and lifewriting to appreciate Annie's entries for their value: they worked against story as a way to keep her alive and sane. Eventually, when my aunt realized that I was serious about working with Annie's diary, she bequeathed me the actual ledger book, a book as thin as Annie herself, binding disintegrating in my hands. Until you hold the past like that, cradle a page where another human being has pressed their own hands, made their mark, asserted the existence of their "I," you might think that old documents are boring or dead. But one of the powers of writing is its ability to transcend time. Annie sat in her claim shanty and wrote about her days, and, more than a hundred years later, I read every word. Her present became my present.

From my work with Annie's diary, I would publish a book based on reading those scant entries and argue for the importance of granting every writer agency and authorship—even if at first their efforts don't seem noteworthy or interesting. No writing, I thought, should be discarded as empty or worthless. Even what I eventually learned to call ordinary writing was extraordinary. Years later, I would turn my gaze to the letters of the American modernist Georgia O'Keeffe and find myself in one of the most prestigious archives in the world—the Beinecke Rare Book and Manuscript Library at Yale—but the feeling of holding the past in my hands would be the same. Here is the paper she chose. Here, the pen. Here, the way her lines loop or wobble. Here, the place she cried.

As we continue to consider ways to generate ideas, I would encourage to try writing from primary materials. My guess would be that you have access to these kinds of documents, even if you don't have access to a university library. Many of us have letters and diaries from our ancestors, often stored in boxes in the basement or in a plastic shoebox on a shelf. Maybe your parents keep them. You might also live near a small local museum or the public library. Ask around. The documents need not be a century old, but the writing exercise I offer below works best when you can physically hold the letter or diary—the actual letter or diary, not a photo or a reproduction or transcription. It's worth doing the leg work to find such a document. Think of it as a first step into research, something all writers undertake. Finally, it doesn't matter whether you know this person—one of your ancestors—or if you have absolutely zero context. I just want you to have the experience of holding the written past in your hands.

Our impulse will be to turn immediately to content, but I would encourage you to delay. Deep seeing always begins with the material, the gross. So take a single page of your written document and examine its physicality. What do you notice about the kind of paper used? Where might that paper come from? Rather than a pre-printed diary available at that time at any five-and-dime, Annie chose a lined ledger book, one that apparently first contained her husband's accounts for his blacksmithing. That matters. Annie had to fit her words into the spaces left over from her husband's "more important" work. She was simultaneously not contained to the number of lines the diary publishers of the time allotted a diarist each day. That's freedom. So when you ask yourself about why the writer chose this paper, you want to also ask yourself what other choices could they have made and what does that tell you about purpose or resources, gender, class, race, literacy, access, and so on.

Make note of imperfections on the page, stains, smudges, bends, and folds. You can never assume the writer is the one to have made the marks—unless you are reading a writer like O'Keeffe who abhorred stains of any kind and would always comment in her letter if she had marred the page—but dirt or smudges show layers of readership. A document from the past has been marked by the world. You want to attend to those imperfections as if they were scars on a body with stories of their own. Before even reading, notice the way the lines move on the page, how they heed or don't heed the margins, whether some lines arrive crossed out (again you cannot assume the writer is the one who is censoring), if the lines run straight or angled, if the hand is cramped or full. What is the feeling you have when you look at the page? Do the lines seem open and flowing or reserved, cautious? These are, of course, just impressions, but we are working from our gut, so we want to trust what arises.

Finally, read the document, a challenge all its own. Most of the primary source material I have encountered in my life does not yield readily. Many of us aren't accustomed to reading long lines of cursive, and handwriting can appear impenetrable. But you just sit with it. See what you can piece together, maybe even start a transcription on the computer. Here is where delight truly arises because you are dipping into the language of the past—words you might not know, syntax that feels foreign, sentiments that can appear overblown and sentimental. Relish all the strangeness. Let the language roll around on your tongue.

Wednesday, April 26, 1882
Clear and Pleasant. Charley got His potatoes and vegetables ready to sell today. I worked hard all forenoon and went to see the Dr this P.M. He put some Nitric Acid on my foot. I am very tired tonight. Charley done up all the work.

You have fallen backward in time. Don't ask the document to live in the twenty-first century. Instead, grant the document its history and the wisdom it offers you. There was once a beating heart beneath every single line. They slanted their page to write. The wick of the lantern turned low, a circle of light amid the dark plains. The palm of their writing hand rested on the blank page below, and they wrote to the sound of their pen as well as an owl calling from a nearby tree. Every letter, every loop, every movement across the page inscribed the presence that you now hold. It is an honor to sit with the writer. Be grateful that they took the time to write, that what they wrote remained, and that you have now added your pulse, your body warmth, your skin cells to this record (record, from the Latin, to take into the heart).

Once you have truly seen what you hold in front of you, once you can close your eyes and envision those lines on your inner eyelids, then open your notebook and begin to write. You can write about the experience of holding the document or you can write about the content expressed. You can generate questions that you want to pursue later. Maybe a character walks into your notebook or a conflict or an entire story. Perhaps you will feel called to write back to the author, a letter of your own. Most often, we have more questions than answers. One letter or one diary entry can begin an entire project (look at what happened when I met Annie Ray). And maybe that will be the case for you. Or maybe what matters most in this writing exercise is that moment when you held the past, when the past took on a shape, a heft, a texture, because maybe that is the very moment you really understood how writing stitches us together, binds us, threads us to those who have been before. And once you realize that, then maybe you humble yourself to the ground when you recognize that the words you place today on the page might not just outlive you but form another's present moment, that your words might possibly be held by hands of the future.

17

Trust the Treasure

Because the writing we do in writing notebooks is low-stakes writing, we might make the error of equating low stakes to low in value—that somehow this writing that we do every day has no value because it may never see the light of day. Nothing could be further from the truth. In fact, return here, if only in your head, to the map you drew of your neighborhood and the five indelible moments that you chose. Maybe even recall the one indelible moment you ultimately selected to explore. Perhaps it has grown into something even larger at this point. Think for a moment about all that had to happen for that one small moment to step forward and offer itself as a subject. If you are in your early twenties, say, you have been on the planet for about 10,000 days. And each of those days has 1,440 minutes. Just consider how many experiences you have had by this point in your life. Millions. Millions of moments. Our brains cannot possibly hold each and every experience. We would explode. Instead, the brain makes decisions all the time about which experiences to store, and for how long, and which to release to the vast annals of the unnarrated. The thinking part of the brain makes that decision only after the moment has passed through what we might call the heart-mind.

In the previous chapter, I pointed out that the word "record" comes from the Latin for heart (*cordis*), as in to carve something into the heart. What we carry as memory, we carry because the heart has determined its value—*not* the head. When we sift back over our day at the dinner table at night, or write in our journals, or as we drift off to sleep, some moments from the day will step forward. For the most part, these moments are attached to an emotion. The more elevated the emotion, the more likely the brain will store the memory. All experiences pass through the "reptilian" part of our brain, the limbic system, and they are *felt in the body as emotion before they become thought*. This is really important. Any experience we have has already been processed by the limbic system. If the limbic system determines there is a reason for the body to be afraid, it activates the sympathetic nervous system and we prepare to fight, flee, or freeze. The body must work this way. Even though thoughts happen in a split second, that split second is long enough for us to die by bear claw or gun.

On a basic level, then, experiences are emotions before they are thoughts. When the emotion is strong enough, then the brain determines that whatever has just happened should be stored. If the experience is a traumatic one, the body stores it in the amygdala, part of the limbic system, and the thinking mind will have no verbal access to that experience—which causes PTSD and we will consider trauma and the body later in the book—but most experiences pass through the limbic system, soaked with emotional resonance, to arrive in the thinking part of our brains and become memories. The more often we recall that memory, the deeper into the brain it burrows (though, and this is fascinating, recent research tells us that every time we recall a memory, we also alter it, so the memory burrows deeper but also travels further away from the "truth"). Here, I just want us to think about what has to happen for us to be able to choose five moments from among millions of experiences and then to narrow to a single moment that we begin to write about. Of the millions of experiences you have had in your life, hundreds of thousands in your childhood neighborhood alone, your brain has stored, say, several thousand. Of those several thousand, when asked, you then selected five. Of those five, you settled on one. One among millions. That you single out this one moment *means* something. That memory has significance. It has dimension and complexity and depth and all the delicious qualities that any writer seeks in their work. By definition. Period. This is the moment that you called up on this particular day. There are no versions of the universe where you can dismiss that memory as unimportant or empty. It may appear, on the surface, to be shallow or uninteresting, but biologically speaking, it can't be meaningless. Your body is telling you to attend. Your brain has not only stored the memory but you have consciously or unconsciously replayed that memory so often that years later, it rises first in your mind.

Trust it. Trust the treasure that you have been offered. It has landed in your lap. On this day. Right there. Trembling in the colors of the past. Your job, as a writer, is to remain with the memory for as long as it takes to figure out why it matters—not why it matters to you personally, though you may begin there, but why it matters to you in your *art*. Memories are moments waiting to be transformed into metaphor. The events that remain with us cannot simply be neutral events from the past. They have been magnified by the emotional state in which they arrived in the physical body. Therefore, they have some deeper message. Your job, as a writer, is to decode the message.

Let me give you an example. When I was in the second grade, I stopped going to school. My mother would drop me off at Fairhill Elementary each morning, and, before lunch, I would be in the nurse's office asking if I could go home. For the first few days, the nurses placated my distress by calling my mother. I was, after all, a "good girl," so they assumed I was telling the truth. When asked, I complained of headache or stomach pain. The nurse would walk me to her office to lie down while I waited for my mother, who would soon enough arrive—conjured by my words, face full of concern, ready to take me home. Later in bed, cozy against the Virginia winter, I would listen as my mother made dinner in the kitchen or played blocks with my toddler brother, the tumble of wood, the shush of faucet, steam from a boiling pot trilling up the stairs. Those afternoons at home are some of the sweetest of my life; I had crossed a threshold to another world, with warmth and rhythm all shaded lemon yellow, the world that existed every day when I was at school learning how to multiply numbers or spell "their."

Within the week, though, everything changed. The doctor could find nothing wrong with my eight-year-old body. The good girl was healthy and perfectly fine. From that moment on, my mother refused to come and get me. I would remain for an entire day in the nurse's dark office. No one would check on me, take my temperature, offer me water. Soon the office itself, a calming den before, was refused to me as well. I was willed back to the classroom, made to be okay.

I learned to stop asking.

In recalling this experience, which lasted maybe a week, I could easily categorize it as just being a kid, my own nuttiness, or a temporary glitch in what would become a perfect attendance record. After all, on first glance, the memory appears already read: a girl fakes illness to avoid going to school. We know that story. But, as a writer, I don't believe any memory is superficial or unimportant. And I certainly don't believe the past has already been read. So I stay with it. I think about what else was happening in my life at the time. I remember that we had only recently moved to Virginia, left the warmth and color of Hawaii for the gray skies of Fairfax County. As a military child, I knew, even at that age, that my duty was to go where the Navy sent us. It's possible that my sickness was the only way I could name a sadness that I was taught to endure. Conscripted by birth, military children are every bit the soldier even if they never don a uniform. In this memory, I see how much I yearned to be cared for—by the nurse, the teachers, my mother—how much I wanted to be home. The emotion attached to the memory is a desperate need to be with my mother. When I sit with that longer, I remember that, close to this same time, my parents left us alone with my grandparents for two weeks while they took a vacation. These were the same years that my grandfather was sexually assaulting my aunt and my cousins, who weren't much older than me. The following summer, he would assault me in a way that I could recall. I cannot tell you what my grandfather may or may not have done to me in those weeks. But I can tell you that the girl I was then sought a tether to her mother and the safety of being inside a brick house. Her need was bone deep and desperate. She would do anything to get home, including lie. The memory begins to pulse with meaning: a child discovering all the ways a body can be betrayed. Now I can write into the past or use my understanding to complicate speakers and characters.

Whether a fiction writer, poet, or nonfiction writer, our job is to trust that what arises when we write about our past has a significance far beyond the superficial. Remember, memory is never neutral. It is charged by emotion. We store these moments from the past because our heart-mind turned them into stepping stones or sign posts, not as a way to remember the experience as data but rather to chart our transformation into the humans we are today. Trust what your body gives you. Trust it every time. And then use what you discover when you turn memory into metaphor to enrich your characters, your speakers, your own wise heart.

18

No One Blames the Baby

When Robin Wall Kimmerer writes in *Braiding Sweetgrass*, "The land is our real teacher. All we need as students is mindfulness," she transforms the earth beneath our feet into our guru. Centuries of resource exploitation in the West, stemming, in part, from Judeo-Christian beliefs that humans hold dominion over the garden, have resulted in the present burning of the earth. Kimmerer finds the root of this destruction in language itself. As an example, she points to the fact that in Western languages the natural world is grammatically assigned to the category of nouns—things that can be acted upon. Native languages, though, often see the nonhuman as verb—agentive and powerful. She writes,

> A bay is a noun only if water is dead. When bay is a noun, it is defined by humans, trapped between its shores and contained by the word. But the verb *wiikwegamaa*—to be a bay—releases the water from bondage and lets it live. "To be a bay" holds the wonder that, for this moment, the living water has decided to shelter itself between these shores, conversing with cedar roots and a flock of baby mergansers. Because it could do otherwise—become a stream or an ocean or a waterfall, and there are verbs for that, too. To be a hill, to be a sandy beach, to be a Saturday, all are possible verbs in a world where everything is alive. Water, land, and even a day, the language a mirror for seeing the animacy of the world, the life that pulses through all things, through pines and nuthatches and mushrooms.

Kimmerer suggests, with her "grammar of animacy," that if we reframe the way we describe the natural world around us, we will be less willing to destroy it because we will see ourselves as connected to it, not separate and above.

One of the wonders of the natural world and one of the great lessons it teaches is that, as far as we know, a tree has never wanted to be a rabbit, nor a rabbit a tree. A tree brings all its bearing, all its energy, its entire being to its "treeness." We should take note, for humans spend most of their days wishing to be something other than they are—younger, thinner, smarter, happier. Most of our suffering arises from our inability to just be, say, "Jennifer," to invest our entire being in our "Jennifer-ness." Rilke speaks to the steadfast ability of nature to honor itself and not yearn to be something else when he writes, "everything in Nature grows and defends itself any way it can and is spontaneously itself, tries to be itself at any and all costs and against all opposition."

The one opportunity we afford humans to be entirely themselves and not ask them to be anything else is when they are babies. No one blames a baby for spitting up on their fresh outfit, or pooping outside their diaper, or crying until they are held. No one blames a baby for anything other than a poor night of sleep. Even then, we know it isn't the baby's fault. We let the baby become, without judgment or punishment, not unlike the way we allow the tree in the front yard to grow or the daisies in the garden to flower. We grant the baby their becoming for a certain number of years, maybe three or four. Usually, with the appearance of language, we begin to assume that the tiny human is no longer freely becoming but rather somehow in charge of their blooms.

This is a tragedy. We are human *beings*, not a human *been*. We are always in the process of becoming. Our heartbeat ushers us ever forward, our cells regenerate, a new day dawns to infinite possibility, and yet we so often chastise ourselves for our failings, our limitations. We want to have arrived or we want a new departure gate. We yearn to be a rabbit.

Nowhere is this more true than in our lives as writers. Every writer I know is plagued by doubt and a sense of inferiority, even the "successful" ones. So especially here, as we focus on generating ideas, we want to treat ourselves as babies, not in the sense of being novices but rather in the sense of being blameless. There is no way to write wrong, just like there is no way to be a tree that is wrong. Your writing is your writing; the tree is the tree. And like the tree, we want to invest ourselves in the process of writing not the arbitrary bar of writer. When we do, we cannot fail. Clouds never fail at their fleecing.

Once when I was rock climbing with Michael in Logan Canyon, I slipped on the cliff face. Even when you know you are safe, falls are jarring. Often you have no warning; your fingers just let go. Because I was on top rope, I didn't swing far, but I still worried about injuring myself on a rock edge or shelf. The rope took me to the right, and I steadied myself where I landed, my heart beating from the fall. I yelled down to Michael to "take" and paused to catch my breath. There, in the limestone in front of me, feet off the route, was a tiny little grotto in the rock protecting three sweet purple asters. They grew as a family in soil I could not see, the morning sun matching their yellow centers. I imagine no human had seen those flowers, unless they had taken the same fall, the same swing. They were simply growing in their grotto four miles up Logan Canyon and fifty feet from the ground. The flowers asked for nothing from anyone. They did not need to be seen. They were content to grow, to become, to thrive, regardless of what was happening in the rest of the world. I keep those flowers with me. They remind me of what it means to live from my heart.

If you happen to be near a window, look outside. Or next time you are walking outside, look around. See if you can find a tree, or a cloud, a bird, or a flower. Just notice its emphatic presence and inherent security, how it is "spontaneously itself." Maybe take a tree or a rock or a bird for your guru. Return to it every time you want to tell yourself a story of failure, lack, or inability. Be like the rock or the bird or the sky and give yourself the gift of your eternal becoming. Allow no one to take your becoming away from you. Insist on your grotto and the way the sunlight bathes your face.

19

The Spellwork of Others

When asked, almost every writer who has ever visited my university has told students that the single most important thing they can do to become better writers is to read. And they don't mean a news feed. They mean deep reading in literary work. But I often wonder if students get scared by that advice, if they worry they don't know what to read or how to read or will somehow do it wrong. I see that fear exposed when they lob canonical authors around the room during a class discussion or shrink when I ask them what books they read over break.

Indeed, most of the writers I know are obsessive readers. They are the ones who read the back of the same cereal box every morning and can list the first four ingredients in Cheerios. They are the ones who scan every poster pasted above the seats of the city bus. When standing in line at the DMV, they pore over the organ donor pamphlet seven times. In *Ex Libris*, the writer Anne Fadiman confesses, "I'd rather have a book, but in a pinch I'll settle for a set of Water Pik instructions." Language is the medium for a writer, just like paint is for a visual artist or wood for a carver. We are interested in all the ways that words can appear, the work they do in the world, how the same words can be cast to sell toothpaste or make us weep.

But when asked to read more intentionally, say, as a writer would read, we can grow nervous. All of a sudden, what you have been doing unconsciously your entire life (sign posted at the elevator, flyer stapled to the telephone pole) fails to qualify as reading and serious reading feels too scary and something best left to teachers.

Here's the thing: you can be a writer who has never read *Finnegans Wake*, a writer who can't articulate how *House Made of Dawn* breaks form, a writer who confuses Wordsworth and Whitman.

It is less what you read and more how you read.

In yoga, there is a practice called *svādhyāya*. Loosely translated, *svādhyāya* means to draw close to something, specifically the self. Historically, the practice of *svādhyāya* (the way one draws close to the self) is through reading, particularly the reading of yogic scriptures. As writers, we can learn a lot about how to read by seeing how yogis have read throughout centuries. First, even though traditionally the texts being read were texts like the *Upaniṣads* or the *Bhagavad Gītā*, sacred lines, there is nothing in the understanding of *svādhyāya*, that says the books have to be holy. They are made holy by our sustained attention. Sri Swami Satchidananda writes that when you practice *svādhyāya*, "anything that will elevate your mind and remind you of your true self should be studied." Elevate the mind. Remind you of truth. He goes on to say that the books you want to read are the books that can't be exhausted by re-reading. He doesn't name those books because he knows that they will differ from person to person. Consider for a moment what poems, essays, novels, or stories ask you to return again and again—either because you love them or because you don't understand them and sense they have something to teach you. What are the inexhaustible reading wells in your life?

Second, Sri Swami Satchidananda lets us know how to approach these books—by "studying with the heart." We don't read to become what he calls "walking libraries," individuals who mine their reading for "logic, quoting, or fighting." We want to read as a way to return to ourselves, not as a weapon to deploy, intimidate, or conquer. Other areas of our life might require that we read in order to argue, but when we read at the start of our writing day, we read to ascend. He compares *svādhyāya* to visiting the Empire State Building. We begin on the ground floor, limited by our view. Each moment spent inspired or challenged or moved by the page before us, we climb higher and begin to see more. At the top, our vision is unlimited. We see our fundamental humanity, our connection, our oneness. In that way, *svādhyāya* becomes, as B. K. S. Iyengar writes in *Light on Yoga*, "the study of one subject which is the basis or root of all other subjects or actions, upon which the others rest, but which itself does not rest on anything."

One final point about *svādhyāya* and that is, Swami Satchidananda reminds us, that you must "put into practice what you read." Our study leads directly to our page. Which is why I am suggesting that you add daily reading, reading as a yogi would, to your practice. Read the inexhaustible, read with your heart, and read always to ascend.

Lastly, one of my favorite witches, the writer Pam Grossman, is always quick to point out the relationship between the spelling of a word and the spell cast by a witch—both transform the gross into the subtle. The letters H E A R T are just letters, but when sorrow arrives at your door, the tearing in your chest swells far beyond the edges of the letter *H*. Grossman also sees etymological connections between grammar and grimoire, a witch's book of spells, which turns the entire system of language into a series of incantations. As writers and artists, we want to embrace the alchemical properties of language—we want to be transformed by our reading and the spellwork of others and then we want to cast our own incantations. If you want to practice *svādhyāya*, here are some guidelines to consider:

- It helps if your daily reading is in a genre other than the one you are writing. A prose writer might read poetry; a poet, short fiction.
- It helps if you choose something brief for your daily reading, something that arrives in a tiny package. Poetry works well but so do letters sent between artists or diary entries. You only need to read for a few minutes before you begin to write. It's nice to select something self-contained, so that you don't have to spend time remembering what has come before. A book like Ross Gay's *The Book of Delights* would be another option.
- It helps to understand that there are sites of reading. We read differently depending on where we are physically. For example, on my bedside table, I keep novels that are fun to read—strong narrative line, interesting setting. That is the reading I do before bed. Its purpose is to entertain. Before meditation, I read a single poem, often Hafiz or Rumi or Kabir. The purpose of that reading is to remind me that I am connected to everything. At my desk, I read other nonfiction writers who are experimenting with form or writing about trauma or reinventing language. I underline, annotate, and study; my reading is much more active. It's helpful to understand where you are reading and why you are reading and to remember that the daily reading you do before you write is there to lift you up.
- Finally, even though it can be challenging, it is helpful to think of your daily reading as a conversation, one you are having with others, some living and some dead. For a conversation to be successful, only one person speaks at a time, and the other person is not simply silently sitting but rather actively listening, trying to really hear what it is the other person is saying. I would encourage to read for companionship on the path and not to find fault and criticize. Remain humble, truly listen, and then, when you are ready, add your voice.

20

Writer's Eyes

In 2015, Pope Francis visited the United States. I remember watching news clips of him moving among the crowds of people who had come out to see him. Young and old alike leaned over the barriers in the streets, hoping to catch a glimpse of the pope as he passed. Almost to the person, they all held cell phones in their hands. Rather than looking at the pope, meeting his eyes, seeing his smile, every single person was fixated on their phone, trying to capture a selfie: "me and the pope."

I can only imagine what the pope's experience that day must have been like—to move into the crowds and have the people literally turn their backs to you. Shepherd to a flock of skulls. Those lining the streets that day probably tell friends and strangers alike that in 2015, they saw Pope Francis. But did they? Bent on documenting their own presence, all of those people blinded themselves.

In yoga, and Hinduism more broadly, there is a concept called *darshan*. It's a kind of mutual or reciprocal seeing. When a pilgrim sees a holy person, they may experience *darshan*, a blessing given to them by the guru or saint simply because of the sighting. The act of seeing, then, is not about the perception or evaluation of the external world; it is about opening oneself to receive the gifts that arise from being seen by it. We, as writers, want to engage in reciprocal seeing. Our traditional understanding of what it means to see is entirely one-directional: the viewer grasps the world with their eyes and then owns it. "I have seen the Grand Canyon," we say. What we mean is that we stood on a spot at the edge of a cliff and spent five minutes gazing across a distance too immense to fully realize, a landscape so vast and varied that our hearts actually started to beat faster, and then we jumped back in the car and now tell people, "I have seen it." When we see this way, when we move through the world as a forager, seizing moments like berries to be consumed, never wondering what we are being offered at the time, never opening to possibility, mutability, and love, we are blinded in two ways. First, we do not see what is actually before us, and second, we then assert that what we have not actually seen is the true, the real, the fixed, the known.

As writers, we want, instead, to meet the world with the eyes of one who walks down the street wanting to be altered, one who knows that the sacred and the holy surrounds us if we only open our eyes. one who looks in order to receive—receive inspiration, receive complication, receive beauty, and, most importantly, receive a truth, which may be messy, mutable, electric, and pulsing. Reciprocal seeing means that we are changed by what we see. We don't see out; instead, the seen enters in.

What would it mean to walk out your door today and believe that every person you met was a holy person, that every person had something to give you if you paused long enough to receive the gift? When we are actively writing, every day, we begin to see the entire world as story or a poem or a narrative. Everything informs our writing. Why? Because we are being offered gifts every single moment of the day. We just have to change our understanding of what it means to see. What is that dandelion growing between the cracks of the sidewalk offering you? What is that cloud that catches at the hem of the mountain asking of you? What is that person standing in front of you at the post office helping you to understand about your essay, your story, your poem?

The whole world is offering itself to us but not as another possession to be owned. The fixed, the stable, the already read and determined, the known: these are all obstacles to the path of a writer. They are obstacles to the path of a human as well. Instead of seeing the world, let the world see you. Let the trees and the sky and the tumble of weeds drifting across the road enter you. Gurus, all of them. When a pilgrim experiences *darshan*, it is like being struck by lightning. No gentle nudge here. When you are seen by the holy, the jolt runs to your toes. The word for this is *shaktipāta*—struck by lifeforce itself.

The last time Michael and I were in India with our children, Aidan and Kellen, we spent a few days in Kolkata. We had come to the city to visit Sri Ramakrishna's ashram on the banks of the Ganges, but while we were there, Michael and I also wanted to visit the Kalighat temple in the middle of town. In one version of the ancient stories, the goddess Parvati shreds her body into pieces because the world is not ready to know her. These bits of flesh fall all over the subcontinent—a finger here, an eye here, a navel here. The site where each piece fell became a holy place where a temple was built to honor that part of the goddess. The right big toe of the goddess landed in Kolkata, and we visited her temple.

India is hot, and Bengal especially hot. The day we arrived, sweat gathered under my arms and at the small of my back. The temple is not set on some grassy slope, away from the city, guarded by rows of banyans. Instead, just like the goddess herself, it's right there in the middle of everyday humanity. Motorcycles and motor rickshaws swarmed in and around the temple. Stalls selling chai, books, and figurines crowded the entrances and exits. We followed the throng as it moved into the grounds and added our bodies to a giant, seething, swerving line of people waiting to receive *darshan* from the temple deity: Kali.

Michael and I tried to remain steady as the line moved forward. Eventually we left the direct sun and entered the dark chambers of the temple itself. While the walls were shadowed, they were not cool to the touch, and the proximity of so many people in a confined space made me feel panicked and scared. Once you are part of that kind of a thrumming, though, there is little chance of leaving. The line accretes into a single body, like a murmur of birds in the sky. We were simply carried along in this wave of humans, moving ever deeper into darkness and the inner sanctum, noise climbing the walls, bells, incense, smashed flowers at my feet. At times, the swell of bodies lifted me from the ground. Then, I was literally carried by a faith in something beyond the physical.

At the moment we viewed Kali herself, a figure covered in flowers, her tongue red with blood, the sound and pressure were so intense that all sense of edges and boundaries were lost to me. I was just in sound, in flesh, in darkness. No outside, no inside. We moved but remained still. I could not tell you whose hand I was holding, whose back I followed, whether my feet remained in the air or on the ground. Kali glowed on the altar. One glimpse, and the sea of humans swept me past. That, to me, feels like *darshan*. For the briefest of moments, I was penetrated by the world.

We will not always be changed by what we see, but we want to engage the world as if we might be. We want to imagine our seeing not as taking but as receiving. The poet Kabir writes, "The Holy one lives inside you—why open your other eyes at all?" Seeing is an offering made by the universe. Let the aster in the crevice whisper what it knows.

21

The Muse Is a Myth

They go by the names of Clio, Euterpe, Thalia, Melpomene, Terpsichore, Erato, Polymnia, Urania, and Calliope. The last is often depicted holding a writing tablet, while the first embraces a scroll. Urania twirls an entire planet on her fingertips. Their father is Zeus and their mother no one other than Memory herself. Collectively, the Muses of ancient Greece have given their names to our modern words "music" and "museum" as well as the verb "to muse," the noun "amusement," and the adjective "amusing." Their role, in the West, as the inspiration for the arts as well as the ancient sciences, has influenced our understanding of the creative process for thousands of years. Many a poet, painter, and potter have attributed their success to the aid of the muses, unseen inspiration from above. Famously, Homer, in the first line of the *Iliad*, invokes the muse: "Sing, O muse, of the rage of Achilles, son of Peleus, that brought countless ills upon the Achaeans." He is not alone.

For many, the idea of divine inspiration provides the only reasonable way to explain how a single human being could create the *Ninth Symphony* or *Nude Descending a Staircase*. How else would a man who cannot hear compose music known the world over? How else could a single artist abstract the human form into motion itself? Certainly that had to come from beyond. Think of the word "inspiration"—literally to have the divine breathe into you, animate you. Deep in our language lies a belief (or hope?) that art arrives from the gods, and, if we pay homage to their presence, they will bless us in turn.

Of course, the hope that our art resides somewhere outside of our own experience becomes a damaging stance for writers—and, more often, a poor excuse for why we do not write. We wait for the muse to arrive before we set pen to page. Ready and willing to open the door if they would only appear, we ultimately shut ourselves off from the true source of craft: *labor*.

Even though most of us would say that we don't actually "believe" in the muse and most of us aren't setting oranges on the altar at their feet, we often act as if the muse is out there by telling ourselves that we aren't ready to write, have nothing to write about, don't feel inspired, or are waiting for the right moment, the right idea, the right conjunction of Jupiter and Saturn. Waiting suggests something is on its way. But we already know there is nowhere to go. It's all right here. Even if we do not name the waiting as muse, we often work with a mindset that looks outside for source.

In addition to the expectation that something must arrive before we begin is another deep-seated belief that, once the muse appears, we become an unfettered channel of creativity and production. Think of someone like Jack Kerouac, who advocated in his "Essentials of Spontaneous Prose" against "selectivity of expression" in favor of "free flowing deviation (association) of mind into limitless blow-on-subject seas of thought." "No revisions" he prescribed as a way to maintain "the purity of speech" so that the moment delivers a "telepathic shock" to the reader. Doesn't that sound pretty nice? Wait for the muse, write with abandon, and never revise. Who wouldn't choose to be consumed by what Kerouac calls "the laws of orgasm" when it comes to craft? Sounds pretty rich.

Except that it's a myth. Literally, it's a myth. Somehow we have forgotten that the Greeks created stories to describe the indescribable not as practical guides for daily life. We choose to do a load of laundry or rearrange our sock drawer because we aren't feeling "inspired" that day. Stephen King, in *On Writing*, says it best:

> Don't wait for the muse. As I've said, he's a hardheaded guy who's not susceptible to a lot of creative fluttering. This isn't the Ouija board or the spirit-world we're talking about here, but just another job like laying pipe or driving long-haul trucks. Your job is to make sure the muse knows where you're going to be every day from nine 'til noon. Or seven 'til three. If he does know, I assure you that sooner or later he'll start showing up.

Writers are no different than masons or plumbers or farmers. They build their lines one word at a time. It's the only way it works. You cannot arrive at the end of the sentence without beginning the sentence. And no one else is going to lay down that pipe for you. Any magic that happens—and I certainly believe in magic—happens because we are at the desk working. The work engenders the mystical, the aha, the epiphany. It's down there in the mud that inspiration resides. Down, not up.

According to Ryan Pelton, Steven Pressfield wears boots to write every day in order to remind himself that labor alone creates fiction. He writes in the muck and mire. The memoirist Christopher Gonzalez tasks himself with 2,000 words every day and will not go to sleep until he has laid each and every one down. Importantly, Gonzalez does not set aside a chunk of time every day to write because his days are too full. Instead, he wedges his 2,000 words in between meetings and teaching and driving his daughters to dance. Gonzalez warns writers not to get hung up with the actual quota. In fact, he reassures, you might decide on 305 words a day, which, on the surface, he says, "is not very much, and you would be right. But if you committed to writing 305 words every day for a year, you would have a manuscript of 111,325 words." The number doesn't matter; the commitment does. I do not know of a single writer who would say that writing is anything but work. And while many, including myself, can describe moments when they were overtaken by a kind of Kerouacian state, those moments happen because you are doing the work. They don't come from outside the work but rather from inside it.

Ultimately, the death of the muse frees us. We no longer wait. We only work. And when that moment of frenzy arrives, that moment you cannot write fast enough because the way forward has become so clear, so pressing, so certain, we understand that we, too, are responsible for that grace as well as all the hours of stagnation that came before. We are the muse. Memory is our mother, and planets spin on our fingertips.

PART TWO

Fullness—*Āntara Kumbhaka*

22

Fullness

We have spent the first part of the book exploring the inhalation, the spring of the breath: generating ideas. In this part, we turn to the fullness of drafting: the building blocks of writing. At the end of my yin classes, my students and I chant the same *shloka* every week. The words come from the *Īśa Upaniṣad*, an ancient text dated by most scholars to the first millennium BCE. Like many revealed truths, the verse appears simple, even flat. The translation of the *pūrṇa* mantra could be rendered: all of this is full; all of that is full; from fullness, fullness comes; take from fullness and fullness still remains. In Sanskrit, the word *pūrṇa* can be translated as full, whole, complete. It evokes images of the full moon or a cup filled to the brim with water. It also refers to our own perfection.

In English, we have words and phrases like "overfilled" and "beyond full," but such states are impossible. Full, by definition, means full. It cannot be added to, nor can anything be taken away from fullness. Fullness is always full. Think of a candle burning steadily. Bring the wick of another candle to the first. The second alights, but the first does not diminish. A full flame will always remain a full flame, no matter how many other candles you light. In yoga, fullness is our birthright, our actual state. We are entirely, completely whole. But, again, we so often fail to see our wholeness. Instead, we think pieces are missing or being withheld.

The top of the inhalation, all that *prāṇa* swirling at our collarbones, brings our attention to the fullness that exists in our lives. It encourages us to trust in the abundance all around us and refuse the narrative of scarcity. Try it here. Return to your breath and find your four- and six-count breathing. Establish that count for several breath cycles, just enjoying the rise and fall of the breath. Often, I envision myself like a wave, lifting from the ocean of *prāṇa* all around me, taking shape, and then returning back to the sea on exhalation. You are one wave of many, sentient beings everywhere rising and falling with each breath, all of us bobbing on an endless ocean.

Now turn your awareness to the inhalation and let it rise up the front of the body slowly. Feel the breath ascend. Here is spring, new beginnings, a tiny stem emerging from rich soil. When you reach the top of the breath, simply pause. Then slowly begin the exhalation back down the body. I say pause here, rather than hold, because you don't want to grasp at the retention of the inhalation. You do not "own" the breath. It has been freely given to you. You never want to grasp for it. Instead, just pause for a beat or two at the top of the breath, feel how the breath parachutes in the body, becoming round and expansive at the top of the lungs. In the pause, just attend to the circulation or the eddying found in the pause, the *prāṇa* gathered for a moment like a cloud or a lake, pooling and swirling. At the point of fullness, you cannot bring more air into your body. (You will find, with practice, that you can add another sip or two when you think you are at fullness to find your complete *antara kumbhaka*.) This is joy. Right here. Abundance. Gratitude. You cannot be more full; you cannot bring more in. You have arrived at the summer of the breath, green and growing things all around you, the days full of light, the sky vaulted above.

Don't stay long. A beat or two. Just long enough to explore the space. Remember, fullness is always there. You don't have to grab anything. If you stay too long in a space of retention the next inhalation will arrive hurried and rushed. You will know you stayed too long because you find yourself gasping. It might be nice to change your inhalation to a count of four, hold for two or four, exhale for four and then inhale again. Think pause at the top, not clamping. Touch the sky and return. Touch the sky and return. Travel in and out of fullness with ease and grace.

One more note about fullness. In Sanskrit, the full moon is *pūrṇimā*, marked by its inability to be more complete. The moon and the sun offer the two primary luminaries that light our sky. Left to our own, we would wake naturally with the sun and allow it to lead us through our days. In the way it waxes and wanes, the moon offers us monthly lessons in both transformation and rebirth. Many connect the moon to the feminine and, more specifically, to the three stages of the Triple Goddess: Maiden, Mother, and Crone. The waxing moon represents the maiden, the full moon, the Mother, and the waning moon, the Crone. Every lunar cycle follows the same evolution, steadily circling through birth, life, death, and rebirth. Viewed from the earth, the moon withers every month, not unlike the body, eventually becoming invisible in the night sky during the Dark Moon, a time of apparent emptiness, darkness, even death. But our perception of diminishment and void is only because of the relationship between the sun and the moon. As we all know, the moon is a reflection of the sun's light, so at the end of the lunar cycle, the sun no longer shines on the moon, but the moon itself has not diminished. It remains full and complete and whole. Only our perception changes. What appears to be empty is actually full.

In writing, drafting is the summer of the breath, the fullness that pours forth once a project has consumed us. But drafting doesn't always feel like that. Sometimes our page still remains blank. Know in those moments that the page only appears empty. It is really full. Trust that the fullness will be revealed with the coming of next light.

23

Dander and Fluff

In the writing process, fullness relates to the more mechanical aspects of craft—how to shape the material you have been generating. Even though this part of the breath is marked by bounty and plentitude, we have to begin small.

I met my husband, Michael, because he offered a free modem over email to the first person in our graduate cohort to claim it. I replied immediately. I have long said that our meeting highlights two of our most fundamental characteristics: Michael is incredibly generous, and I love a deal. Our first date involved a canoe trip down the Huron River in Michael's heavy aluminum canoe, herons guiding us the entire time. We let the swollen river take us, the paddle less an oar and more a rudder; the moment we pulled the canoe ashore I wanted to do it all again. The natural world, rather than the clink of silver in a restaurant or the sorrowful sound of violin filling a concert hall, would form the backdrop not just of our dates but of our lives. We are, fundamentally, our best selves when we are together in nature, whether fording a river or cresting the saddle of a mountain.

Maybe because Michael spent his early years roaming a forest outside Cincinnati with his older brother or maybe because he was partially raised by an aunt who taught him how to attend, Michael feels increasingly at home the further he moves from crowds and the built environment. Nothing pleases him more than to face a challenge posed by the weather, an errant path, or a boulder blocking a trail—nothing except maybe the joy of making fires. It's primal, the pleasure that a well-made fire gives him, something about the ring of warmth and protection cast by flames. I have basked near countless fires made by Michael in the past twenty-five years, fires built on snow, in sleet, amid rocks, against wind, on sand, prairie, edge of cliff, fires built in the driving rain. What he will tell you about making fires is that you always begin small.

Small for Michael means smaller than twigs. If he is making a fire that he knows must catch—because Aidan and Kellen and I are freezing or wet or hungry—even though time is precious, rather than reach for sticks and small limbs, he actually moves in the opposite direction, to moss and the fuzz that catches in weeds. Once he has lit a tiny ball of fluff on a space swept as clear as possible, he coddles the young flames, cups his hands in protection, waits to see each strand of moss, each tiny hair, glow orange. Only then does he reach for twigs as thin as toothpicks.

Which is why when I gather wood for Michael, I know to return bearing small limbs but also dander and fluff. I lay what I have collected in piles of similar size, and it's always the small pieces that pile high. In all these years, I have yet to see Michael fail to make a fire, but I have also never seen him work from anything other than bits. Patience builds the fire, as well as the knowledge that everything begins with nothing.

Writing works the same. If you recall, Anne Lamott keeps a one-inch picture frame on her desk to remind her to look through the smallest of windows. The great novels of our time, the epic poems, the works that live from one generation to the next, all began with a single word, a single idea, a single image. While the writer may have had some sense of where they wanted to eventually head, they had to actualize that vision by starting with fluff and dander. And that's only good news because all too often the idea of a big project can overwhelm us to the point of paralysis. The title of Lamott's book, *Bird by Bird*, is a reference to this very idea: that we take things one step at a time.

Let's say you'd like to write about your mother, a woman who is complicated. If your friend's mother had warm chocolate chip cookies waiting for them the moment they stepped off the school bus, your mother greeted you at the door with anger or tears, if she greeted you at all. Still, though, you love your mother and knew, even as a child, that she was doing her best. Your relationship is thorny and messy and hard: the kind of material that will burn hot and fierce if you can just find a way to contain it.

You spend a few days writing in your writer's notebook. You cull through pictures, talk with your sister, track down the diary you kept at the age of nine; still, when you sit down to write, all you can register is a general sense of nausea in your belly. You close your laptop, call it a day, and maybe decide to write about unicorns instead.

Or you try again.

Except this time you remember to work small. You don't try to recall that time at the age of sixteen when she locked you outside during a January blizzard or the phone call from the neighbor to inform you that the police were at your house. You don't try to summarize fifteen years of drama in three paragraphs or even three pages. You gather some moss.

The bathroom is where you begin. Sitting on the closed toilet seat watching your mother apply mascara, how she leaned her body close to the mirror, pulled the brush along her lashes as if petting a butterfly. She wore a pink slip as well as purple fuzzy slippers on her feet. The cat curled beneath the radiator, tail covering her nose. Then you move even smaller and remember her hands, how they pulled the powder puff along her cheekbones, how the powder concealed the dark rings gathered under her eyes. Those were the same fingers that traced your face at night in the darkness when you woke from a bad dream, the fingers that sang you back to sleep at a time in your life when monsters under the bed were your only fear. Stay in that bathroom. Let your mother speak. Recall the smell of Ivory soap and the warm, wet air released by the heater. What color were the walls? What about the tile on the floor? Did your mother curl her hair or roll it? Or did she straighten her hair within an inch of its life using a flat iron? See how still she becomes when she adds eyeliner or outlines her lips in pencil? Watch how practiced she is in the way she flicks the hairbrush. Remember the sting of that same brush on the backs of your legs when you were a smart-ass to her. Don't go there yet—just recall. You could live your life in that bathroom. Everything you need or want to say about your complicated, messy, all-too-human mother can be found within those walls. Build the fire there. Protect what you are making. Be patient. If you reach too quickly for something more, what you have will go out.

It's magic or it's just the process. You can decide. But it works. Whether writing a sonnet, a novella, or a family history, you must begin small. If for no other reason, you must start small so that if, and when, the fire does go out, you know how to begin again.

When Michael builds a fire, he always provides the fire "something to aspire to," a single log, which he usually places on top. The log is never large enough or heavy enough to vanquish the flames. In writing, we typically find those logs within the piece itself. Were I to continue working on the scene in the bathroom, I might follow the hairbrush and the knowledge of its shape held by my thighs. Or I might consider her curls, the need to domesticate the wild. Writing generates writing—creates its own sticks to which it can then aspire and move. That is how you build a story or an essay. Begin small, stay small, work small, and follow the sticks that appear. Eventually, you have a bonfire, one capable of warming all that want to gather around. But you cannot get there unless you gather strands and strips and strings and fluff. Like a seed, they contain all.

24

Everyone Gets Naked in a Scene

Simply put, scenes are the amino acids for prose writers (poets, too, when they are working more narratively). They are one of the most important craft elements that a writer learns to develop, and, quite honestly, the one I see most of my students try to avoid. Writers typically avoid writing scenes because they realize, early on, that scenes are hard to write. Painstaking even. (An aside here: for decades, I thought painstaking etymologically related to the staking of pain. But I came to learn, in writing this chapter, that it comes from the taking of pains. Willingly assuming a burden or even a sorrow. I offer the aside to demonstrate how I work as a writer—when I allow myself to stop and research and what that research yields. Here, I come to find that a scene is painstakingly hard to write because it requires a willful acceptance of hardship, even sacrifice.) So scenes are hard. But why?

The more I read and write, the more I understand that many of the choices we make in writing have to do with time and the experience of time. I write more about time and its relationship to form later, but for now I want to think about how the reader experiences time in terms of scene and summary. In the next section, I describe the work of summary, which is generally the long shot, cinematically speaking, where time moves quickly for the reader. A scene does the opposite. It slows time down for the reader. In fact, a scene unfolds in actual time. We move through the scene *with* the characters as they move through the scene. The scene, then, is the present moment, even when written in the past or the future. The reader experiences a scene as unfolding right before them.

A scene is typically signaled by a time peg that lets the reader know they are about to enter a scene: "One day …," "Last night …," "Two weeks later …," and so on. When a reader arrives at such a time peg, they know, intuitively, unconsciously, that they are about to be *shown* something. Readers are savvy. They have been reading for a long time. They read, like writers write, from the gut—meaning, they aren't thinking about what they read but instead are *inside* what they read. John Gardner famously writes that the goal of fiction (his focus is fiction but his point extends to all prose) is a "continuous and vivid dream." For the most part, we want our readers to enter our work and never lift their heads. Readers know what that dream feels like; it's why they read. They want to go on the journey and intuitively understand how prose moves: when cued, they prepare to settle and watch a scene unfold. As the writer, you must deliver.

To be more direct: when a scene begins a reader is expecting to learn something. Otherwise, why have we slowed down? Which means that something important needs to happen in the scene and it needs to happen early on. We want to begin a scene close to the climax of the scene. Scenes are tiny bonfires in prose—burning, burning, burning. The reader does not want to spend time looking for the matches or some kindling. They expect the scene to be on fire from the start.

While a scene is aflame in terms of tension, it is slow in the way it reveals that tension. Again, a scene happens in real time. This means scenes often include dialogue, the characters talking with one another. A scene also requires lots of strong physical detail. Too often writers initially compose scenes that appear to happen in a vacuum. A conversation floating in space. Readers want to see the kitchen, sit at the table, watch the father and son crumble over French toast. I will write more about significant detail and its relationship to scene later. Here, I just want to highlight that there is a physicality to scene work. Bodies acting in the world.

Again, a time peg heralds the beginning of a scene, the reader prepares to slow down and be shown something, the writer begins as close to the burning as possible, and then the writer patiently, patiently, patiently lets the characters interact. Because a reader arrives at a scene and expects something to happen, *something must happen*. The flipside of this maxim is true as well: if it is important to the narrative, then it must happen in scene. We cannot have the murder occur offstage. The reader will leave us. So if we are in scene, then something is happening. If something is happening, it needs to be in scene.

A scene is its own little terrarium. Self-contained. It has its own beginning, climax, and end. Generally speaking, a writer offers a scene in order to complicate what has happened earlier in the narrative. A scene adds a twist or a turn or a further deepening. If we don't move toward increasing complexity with our scenes, then the narrative remains flat and boring. The reader will feel as though nothing is happening, and we will have lost our tension. So scenes build. They have their own tiny narrative arcs. And the reader craves scenes because the scene allows the reader to see the characters "unfiltered." The characters are showing us exactly who they are—how they move their bodies, how they express themselves in language, the way they bite their nails—and then, as readers, we get to decide how to think about that. Summary, exposition, and musing all feel more "filtered" because the reader knows that the narrator is summarizing or generalizing or commenting. In a scene, everyone is naked.

Which brings me to one last point about scenes. To say a scene arrives aflame does not then mean something terrible must happen in scenes. The most terrifying infernos, quite honestly, in both life and art, are the ones where nothing seems to happen. An unstable character eyeing the paring knife left on the kitchen counter is ten times more haunting than him actually brandishing it. A mother need only hold that brush as she straightens her hair. She need not use it on a child's thigh. Scenes can be quiet. Scenes can be soft. But scenes cannot be random. Readers know when a scene begins that something is about to be revealed. It's a compact made between writer and reader, unconscious but body deep. You must show your reader something and you must do it slowly, close up, in real time. Writers will try and cheat all the time by writing in summary because—as we now understand—building a scene is the willful acceptance of burden. Again readers are savvy. They won't let you get away with it. Write the scene.

In conclusion, I offer the start of a scene from Jhumpa Lahiri's short story "Mrs. Sen's." The story centers on a woman, Mrs. Sen, who has recently moved to the United States from her home in Kolkata because her husband has taken a job. Mrs. Sen cannot drive and spends much of her time indoors and alone. Early in the story, she begins to babysit a boy named Eliot, who comes to her apartment. Their time together reveals Mrs. Sen's alienation and sadness. Toward the end of the story, Mrs. Sen decides to try and drive. This is just the beginning of a scene that continues for several pages (in general, scenes should last beyond a single page—which means you need to pick your scenes carefully—you won't have many). Notice the time peg, the physical details, and the dialogue. In a scene, you want every single line to carry more than just description. We assume a burden when we write a scene, but the scene assumes an even greater burden in terms of what it must carry in the narrative.

> One afternoon a few days later the phone rang. Some very tasty halibut had arrived on boats. Would Mrs. Sen like to pick one up? She called Mr. Sen, but he was not at his desk. A second time she tried calling him, then a third. Eventually she went to the kitchen and returned to the living room with the blade, an eggplant, and some newspapers. Without having to be told, Eliot took his place on the sofa and watched as she sliced stems off the eggplant. She divided it into long, slender strips, then into small squares, smaller and smaller, as small as sugar cubes.
>
> "I'm going to put these in a very tasty stew with fish and green bananas," she announced. "Only I will have to do without the green bananas."
>
> "Are we going to get the fish?"
>
> "We are going to get the fish."

"Is Mr. Sen going to take us?"

"Put on your shoes."

They left the apartment without cleaning up. Outside it was so cold that Eliot could feel the chill on his teeth. They got into the car, and Mrs. Sen drove around the asphalt loop several times. Each time she passed by the grove of pine trees to observe the traffic on the main road. Eliot thought she was just practicing while they waited for Mr. Sen. But then she gave a signal and turned.

The accident occurred quickly.

25

Designate a Driver

If scenes are the close-ups in prose, then summary provides the wide angle. The reader stands farther away from the action in summary and time moves more quickly. Think about the camera hovering above a neighborhood at the start of a film, allowing the viewer to see the general layout of the streets, the trees and the houses, the numbers of people out walking or playing on sidewalks. The viewer is afforded a general sense of the time period, the weather, socioeconomic status, and even relative sense of safety. Context is provided by summary as well as background that might be necessary, information we might need before we find ourselves, once again, in scene.

The writer Bill Roorbach in *Writing Life Stories* says it best. He writes that scenes are where the party takes place. They are exciting and dramatic, colorful and blooming with sensory detail. We all want to be at the party because we know that's where everything is happening. If we stay home, we will miss the moment the basketball captain manages to limbo. However, for us to make it from one party to the next, we need a designated driver. Summary is our designated driver. It is summary that tells us when it's time to leave, summary that makes sure we arrive at the next party in good shape, summary that will ultimately drive us home at the end of the night. That metaphor may appear to cast summary as the boring one, but if that's your take on the role of the designated driver, then my guess would be you have never relied on a sober friend. They exist to make sure your story continues.

Summary is not without its bit of glamor. Even the designated driver will dress for the party and look great holding their glass of seltzer. Summary is not without detail, not without specificity, but its role is to move the reader along. Remember, the relationship between scene and summary is a relationship of time. Scenes slow a reader down and summary speeds the reader up. One is not boring and devoid of lyricism, while the other one is flinging Mardi Gras beads. Instead, they work together to control pace.

Given that scenes are where the party happens, you would think that most writers fail to remember to include summary, but, as I wrote in the previous chapter, scenes are hard to write and most writers try to get away with too much summary. No reader, though, will be content to hover above a neighborhood for the length of a short story. The reader wants to move down into the action, see what everyone is wearing, what they are saying, what items they packed into their purse that morning. As writers, we want to find a balance between scene and summary, knowing that scenes unfold in real time while summary moves narrative along. Art is not math, but in general you can aim for seventy percent of your work to arrive in scene with thirty percent holding the other seventy together through summary. Some writers have trouble recognizing when they are writing in scene and when they are writing in summary. Take a highlighter to your page, or use the highlight function on your computer, and literally mark yellow where you are in scene—characters speaking and moving in real time and typically heralded by a time peg—and green when you are in summary—long shot, general overview, passing quickly through time and space. Look at your pages. You want to see a canary, not a prairie.

Again, art is not math, and there may be all sorts of crazy cool reasons you want to remain longer in summary. But you don't want to remain in summary with the hope the reader won't notice. The reader always notices.

While writers tend toward summary because scenes are hard to write, they also rely too much on summary because they are trying to incinerate entire trees rather than the moss and fluff. It's not uncommon for a writer to simply take on too much. Let's say you are writing a short story about a teen who decides to enlist in the military after 911 and then goes to Iraq where he becomes disillusioned by his country's call to arms. You can see the scene in Iraq, the one where the protagonist's friend steps on an IED while checking for children left behind, but to get there you need to tell the reader about the protagonist's relationship with his father, then what happened in Boy Scouts, then how his sister got pregnant at sixteen and chose to keep the baby, but then how the baby had a learning disability, and how the sister lost her job, and then the long nights watching MMA and feeling envy swell for those with a way to land their anger on another body. So you write fifteen pages of summary, giving the reader everything they need to understand about why the protagonist weeps when the nurse hands him the tiny plastic elephant his friend carried in his cammies, but by now the reader has left you. They stopped reading on page three because none of the questions they asked were ever addressed. A pregnant sister? Are they close? What exactly did the Scout leader do? And where is the mother? You were moving too quickly because you needed to get to Riyadh. You may arrive in the desert, but the reader has put down your story in favor of one about a hula dancer.

Summary cannot carry a story. Its role is to get the reader from one scene to the next. Without summary, scenes lose their relationship to one another; they drift. In addition to connecting scenes together, summary can take the reader through large tracts of time and space And the reader craves those moments as well—the times where they step outside the claustrophobic grip of a scene and take a much needed breath. Think about leaving a noisy bar or a crowded restaurant and meeting a dark January sky. Think of how the cold air clamps your body and the silence gathers like a muff around your ears. Think about how, when the door latches behind you, all the jostling and yelling and dancing and laughing disappear. Think of the quiet walk back to the car, your sober friend not talking but just jangling the keys in her pocket. Feel the snow-covered trees around you, the stars so crisp and certain. Feel yourself expand with that pause, that relief. Summary works the same way. We do not want to remain in the bar. We need the walk back to the car.

Below is the summary that precedes the scene from Lahiri's "Mrs. Sen's." Notice how the summary serves to reveal Mrs. Sen's skill and artistry, while also letting the reader know about her relationship with Eliot. We move quickly through time, but the summary is full of detail and frames what is to follow. Still, notice your feeling as you read summary. Consider how long you would be content to move at this pace before you would want to settle down and see the characters interact.

> He especially enjoyed watching Mrs. Sen as she chopped things, seated on the newspapers on the living room floor. Instead of a knife, she used a blade that curved like the prow of a Viking ship, sailing to battle in distant seas. The blade was hinged at one end to a narrow wooden base. The steel, more black than silver, lacked a uniform polish, and had a serrated crest, she told Eliot, for grating. Each afternoon Mrs. Sen lifted the blade and locked it into place, so that it met the base at an angle. Facing the sharp edge without ever touching it, she took whole vegetables between her hands and hacked them apart: cauliflower, cabbage, butternut squash. She split things in half, then quarters, speedily producing florets, cubes, slices and shreds. She could peel a potato in seconds. At times she sat cross-legged, at times with legs splayed, surrounded by an array of colanders and shallow bowls of water in which she immersed her chopped ingredients.
>
> While she worked, she kept an eye on the television and an eye on Eliot, but she never seemed to keep an eye on the blade.

26

There Is No Beethoven

If you were a tailor, scene and summary would be your needle and thread: the most basic tools of your trade, eminently versatile and ultimately irreplaceable. The scene punctures the moment and summary threads those scenes together to create what is sometimes called "profluence," a term coined by John Gardner to describe the way fiction moves forward to either a point of conclusion or exhaustion. For Gardner, profluence applies both to the smooth movement forward within the story and the reader's experience of the story. We want to see what will happen next, so we keep reading. Scene and summary stitch a seam, of sorts, to follow, and their relationship to time allows them to jointly control the pace. When scene and summary are working well together, the reader does not notice where one ends and another begins. Just as you do not question the seams in your pants. You just put them on.

In memoir writing specifically, and nonfiction more generally, a writer can rely on a third element of narrative craft called musing. Fiction writers, as well as poets, also make use of the musing voice, but memoirists *always* make use of it. The musing or reflective voice is just what it sounds like: a place in the narrative where the narrator steps forward to ponder and consider. And just like with scene and summary, musing is related to time, though in a slightly different way. When the narrator steps forward to consider what is happening, it is the I-now narrator looking back at the I-then. For example, Edward P. Jones begins his short story "The First Day" in this way: "In an otherwise unremarkable September morning, long before I learned to be ashamed of my mother, she takes my hand, and we set off down New Jersey Avenue to begin my very first day of school." The fiction writer Amber Caron shares Jones' story with her students when she is teaching them about retrospective narrators. The narrator, a young girl, who narrates the story begins in the I-now. She knows that she will become ashamed of her mother with her darned socks and inability to complete forms, but the girl walking down the street, the I-then, has no idea. The tension between the I-now and then I-then generates dramatic energy, and we read to experience, maybe even resolve, that tension.

In "A Sketch of the Past," Virginia Woolf defines the I-now and the I-then. Woolf describes the I-now as the narrator who writes from the "platform" of the present. They know what will happen to their child self because they have lived their life. The child self, the I-then, does not know and moves through their scenes in a kind of ignorance. The I-now can shape an understanding of the past for the reader in a way that the I-then will never be able to access. This creates dramatic irony—as readers, we know what the I-then will never know. In acknowledging how both the I-now and I-then are constructions of the author, Woolf writes, "I suppose that my memory supplies what I had forgotten, so that it seems as if it were happening independently, though I am really making it happen." Importantly, it is what the I-now comes to understand about the past—about events that may even have been forgotten—that generates meaning beyond what is actually happening on the page. The I-now has a wisdom, a perspective, about the shape of their life. Standing on that tall platform of the present, the I-now sees far beyond the edges of their own story. Woolf writes:

> Perhaps this is the strongest pleasure known to me. It is the rapture I get when, in writing, I seem to be discovering what belongs to what; making a scene come right; making a character come together. From this I reach what I might call a philosophy; at any rate it is a constant idea of mine; that behind the cotton wool is hidden a pattern; that we—I mean all human beings—are connected with this; that the whole world is a work of art; that we are parts of the work of art. *Hamlet* or a Beethoven quartet is the truth about this vast mess that we call the world. But there is no Shakespeare, there is no Beethoven; certainly and emphatically there is no God; we are the words; we are the music; we are the thing itself.

Woolf's assertion that "behind the cotton wool is hidden a pattern" is what makes the musing found in memoir or the retrospective narrator/speaker so compelling for a reader. The I-now can see the pattern that the I-then never will, and the pattern, importantly, is one that the reader recognizes and potentially has experienced themselves: shame, joy, fear, loneliness, and so on. Woolf writes that, once a writer finds the pattern through their awareness of I-now and I-then, they tap into the "truth about this vast mess that we call the world." An experience may be singularly experienced but is ultimately shared. Musing, I would argue, is what frees memoir from solipsism and navel gazing because the I-now is having to come to terms with what has happened and make meaning out of the past. As the I-now suffers alongside the I-then, compassion is born.

As you can imagine, the musing voice is difficult to cultivate. Used with a heavy hand, it feels as if the reader is being told what to think. If preachy and didactic, musing suggests the writer doesn't trust their scene work to convey their ideas. Too much musing can also deny the reader the mystery of discovery, which is one of the primary reasons that we read. When musing is deployed well, though, the story, essay, or poem leaves the realm of dramatic action and moves toward the deeper subjects that bind us together as human beings.

To conclude, I offer a few of the early sentences in my memoir *Ordinary Trauma*. As I write above, memoirists always rely on the musing voice; it's a hallmark of the genre. In this chapter, I am describing what it was like to live on Pearl Harbor as a child. I have begun in summary to establish time period and geographical location, but at the end of the first paragraph the "I-now" steps forward.

> As a child, I was only dimly aware that the oily-black water lapping at my feet concealed an unknown number of bodies and sunken ships. I walked past the concrete memorials with their bronze plaques, traced my fingers along the raised lettering.
> In my yard, bushes dipped and bent in the offshore breezes, oleander and plumeria, hedges of hibiscus and ti, coconut palms, date, mango trees with leaves that glinted like a thousand mirrors. And the flowers: electric pinks, reds, and purples of hanging torch ginger, heliconia, jacaranda, bird of paradise. Bougainvillea climbed the house, the lanai, the tennis court fence nearby. Standing beneath the white plumeria in the corner of my yard, I thought the world perfumed and vibrant, a festival of birdsong.

The I-now, writing from the platform of the present, sees the inherent contradiction found in a childhood spent among bougainvillea and naval destroyers; the I-then plays on a tire swing hung next to a bomb shelter. The I-then doesn't see the paradox. Instead, she wonders what's for dinner. She is forever swinging. The musing voice points the reader toward the tension, which then gets amplified as the scene continues through verbs like "buried" and "amputated" as well as an image of a Chinese banyan too tired to tend its roots. The I-then saw festival and color; the I-now wonders about a peace secured by violence and how such messages infiltrated the domestic space. Importantly, the reader does not have to have lived on Pearl Harbor or have grown up in the military. Musing points to the deeper subjects that bind us all together. In this case, ordinary trauma.

27

Breathing with Caesar

Not unlike Woolf, the great conductor Leonard Bernstein also saw his art as a way to merge with the larger world around him. In an interview with Jonathan Cott, Bernstein says, "If I don't become Brahms or Tchaikovsky or Stravinsky when I'm conducting their works, then it won't be a great performance." In his words, we see Woolf's assertion that we are all Beethoven, that art, just like yoga, has the ability to transcend space and time, to dissolve boundaries between here and there, now and then, you and me.

Breathing works the same way. Literally. As Sam Kean writes in *Caesar's Last Breath*, with every inhalation we take in molecules exhaled by Caesar when he died on the floor of the Roman senate at the hands of his friend Brutus in 44 BCE. His last breath, Kean says, "contained around 25 sextillion (25,000,000,000,000,000,000,000) molecules," which would have entered the atmosphere and circulated only to be ingested again and again and again. Every day, you breathe Caesar thousands of times. Kean writes, "across all that distance of time and space, a few of the molecules that danced inside his lungs are dancing in yours right now." And not just Caesar's last breath, Kean continues, but also the last breath of Jesus, or those at Pompeii, or Jack the Ripper's victims, the last dinosaur, your dead grandmother, or "anything that ever breathed, from bacteria to blue whales."

Every inhalation, then, connects us not just to every sentient being on the planet who is also inhaling, but to every being who has exhaled before us. We are all, in part, mastodon.

Sometimes, I find it hard in my own practice to remember how profound each inhalation and exhalation is. Often one part of my mind is counting my exhalation, while another is running an errand or composing an email. I can practice without actually practicing, which, of course, is not practice at all. When I feel my mind wandering and I sense that my breathing is mundane, I remember something else I heard once about Bernstein. He said that before he conducts a great symphony, he always reminds himself that someone in the audience will be hearing that symphony for the very first time and someone will be hearing it for the very last time. When he thinks of a performance this way, the stakes become much higher.

We can apply the same awareness to our breath on the days when we feel like nothing is happening in our practice, that our breath is unmagical, our writing nonexistent, the gray skies endless. At that point, I return to my inhalation and I remind myself that with that one inhalation I am inhaling at the same time a newborn baby is taking its very first breath somewhere on this planet. And then, when I exhale, that I am exhaling in time with someone who is taking their very last breath. My breath, then, welcomes a new being into the world and serves as a companion to one who is leaving their body behind. We breathe in rhythm with birth and death itself. While we will never know the specific person our breath welcomes or departs with, some day each of us will leave on the exhale, and what would it mean to know that in the world someone was taking that exhalation with us?

I invite you to try this practice the next time your own breath work feels worthless or silly. Or when you feel bored or just tired. Or when your mind keeps chasing down your list of things to do. Instead, take the next inhalation as if it were your first, in unison with another whose lungs fill with air for the very first time. The breath, like art, connects us to all who have come before as well as to the present moment. Breathe with Caesar and Morrison and King. Breathe with Woolf and Mozart and the soldiers missing in action in the War in Vietnam. Breathe with the mastodons and those who etched them into rock. Breathe with the 6,667 women who had to live until child-bearing age for you to take this birth as a human. Truly a miracle. Breathe with the baby who just now entered the world, coated in vernix and blood, pure and perfect.

28

Enter Snake

Ryan Van Meter has a powerful essay entitled "First." I teach it regularly in my introductory classes because it demonstrates in a very short space some of the key craft elements that transmute words into art. Van Meter's essay begins and ends in the back of his parent's station wagon—a "place that feels like a secret"—where he and his friend, Ben, look out the back window while their parents drive home from an outing. The fathers in the front are engaged in traditionally masculine activities—specifically, listening to a baseball game on AM radio—while the mothers chat in the middle seat. Van Meter, though, looks in the opposite direction and takes Ben's jam-sticky hand in his own before leaning in to whisper to Ben that he loves him. The confession of his five-year-old heart stops the car, if not literally, then metaphorically. The radio goes silent. Conversation halts. Van Meter's mother turns her face, "laugh lines not laughing," and forces him to repeat what he has just said. When he does, she responds, "You shouldn't have said that," and returns her son to the dark, to "the tail of the car" that "suddenly feels so wrong."

"First" is a small piece that I have made even smaller in summarizing. Van Meter weaves in moments from the past that help us understand what he has been taught by the larger culture about whom he can love and how. When the mother swivels her head and makes him repeat his confession, the reader understands just how closets get built, then locked. Van Meter is able to point to the ways heteronormativity and beliefs in masculinity destroy a child, destroy him, without ever naming such forces directly. Instead, Van Meter relies entirely on detail.

Significant detail, like musing, moves a piece of writing toward a deeper subject. The magical powers of significant detail to transform the mundane to the pulsing cannot be overstated. Too often, new writers feel they need to write about the dramatic, the emphatic, the gigantic, when really all they need to do is take a look at the objects rolling around at the character's feet.

For Van Meter, both a bat and a set of jumper cables join him and Ben in the backseat. We, as readers, are made aware of both by the third paragraph: "Coiled beside my legs are the thick black and red cords of a pair of jumper cables" as well as Ben's bat, "rolling around and clunking." Now Van Meter is writing nonfiction, so he is bound by the truth. He can't just make stuff up. Both the fiction writer and the poet have more latitude in what they might find in their backseats, but containers for an artist, constraints, are actually helpful in the making of art. We would think complete freedom is what we want, but actually borders and boundaries promote creativity. So, here, in writing his essay, Van Meter is contained by the truth of what was in the backseat of the station wagon. My guess would be that other objects also littered the floor, maybe an empty Coke can or a gym bag or the comic book he brought with him for the ride. Van Meter does not give us those details. He controls our gaze: baseball bat and jumper cables.

A detail becomes a significant detail when it points toward the deeper subject of a piece. Like any detail worth its page space, a significant detail must be a sensory detail, meaning it must activate one of our sense organs. Because we are *Homo sapiens*, with eyes at the front of our heads, visual details are the details we tend to value the most. But a significant detail can and should also elicit the sense of smell or taste or touch. Bats and jumper cables are familiar objects, and their cultural pervasiveness means that most readers will automatically generate an image of each. If they are older readers, their mental image may be a wooden bat; a younger reader might imagine a metal alloy. Doesn't matter. What matters is that the reader see the bat and the jumper cables.

Most details in a piece of writing—especially poetry and flash forms where every word counts—need to pull double duty. It's just not enough that they physically describe a kitchen or a swing set or the entrance to a roller coaster. They need to become significant details where they both describe but then also push toward deeper subject. Van Meter is aware of that in "First," which is why he offers the details that he does. A bat, as a traditional symbol of masculinity as well as the white, middle-class, apple-pie vision of America, trembles with meaning at the feet of a boy who is never going to be straight. If nothing else, it signals the distance between his seat and his father's in the front. More to the point, bats have been used to beat people, people who look different or believe differently or who just don't conform. It is a threatening force rolling around in the back; this bat that "should" be Van Meter's source of play is far from neutral. It marks distance; it lurks; it suggests, at the very start of the essay, that someone is going to be hit.

The jumper cables too are not a random detail that Van Meter grabbed out of thin air; they, too, vibrate. They sit "coiled" right next to Van Meter's leg, snakes waiting to strike. An empty Coke can would point the reader in a different direction or maybe no direction at all. Coil some jumper cables at the feet of a five-year-old who is about to "sin" and a snake enters the garden. A soul is up for grabs in the back of the station wagon, as well as punishment for "sinning."

I know that some of you might say I am reaching too far, that Van Meter meant none of that. I can only speak from experience. As a writer, I am fully aware at every moment of what I am choosing to push forward and what I am leaving unsaid. Details can appear to be superficial or known, but they often need to simmer in a reader's subconscious. Writing is a made thing. One word at a time. And the writer is in charge of the making. If they want to explore larger questions about how we are taught to love, and they want to explore those questions in messy, complicated ways—rather than just rant about their own opinion—then they must rely on the power of significant detail. Give the reader a bat and a coiled snake and the reader understands all that threatens that five-year-old. The violence will not only come from his well-intentioned but scared parents. The violence is systemic and historical and deep. We, as readers, arrive at that understanding through two simple objects—the bat and the jumper cables. What initially appears concrete is allowed to transform.

29

No Dead Grandmothers

A few years ago, I was having a phone conversation with the two women who run the literary agency that had just taken my work. We were discussing the novel I had sent them. Though the three of us had already communicated over email, this was the first opportunity I had to hear their voices and walk with them through the manuscript. While I had expected them to ask for revisions, I realized very quickly that what they wanted to talk about were the characters in the novel, specifically the mother, Lynn. At the end of the novel, it is unclear whether Lynn's marriage will survive. She has reconciled with her teenage daughter, but her husband, a naval officer, remains at sea. For me, the novel ended with the final word. As a writer, I was most concerned with the last image, whether it was too pat, too trite, whether it brought the book toward closure without suggesting that everything would be fine. But the two literary agents were concerned, in large part, with what happened after the novel ended. They asked me if Lynn was going to leave her husband, if Lynn was going to pursue her art, if Lynn had any chance at happiness.

As a memoirist, I am used to readers asking after the health of my father or my mother or my younger brothers. They have sat at the kitchen table with my family, spent months in a Winnebago with them, know the order of states in which we were stationed. If readers have a chance to meet my parents in person, they often begin by saying they feel like they already know them. Readers certainly will say that to me when they meet me, right before they give me a hug. I am always honored by their feelings of connection, though also a bit uncomfortable. The intimacy they experience is both real—I write as vulnerably as I can—but also not real—I have never met them before in my life. Still, I understand that, because I write about my life and those in my life, people will assume they know me or a version of me. This is humbling.

I didn't, though, expect such investment to happen with my fictional characters. So I was surprised when I found myself responding, after a few moments of thought, that Lynn would most likely get divorced. Having lived in Lynn's body for so long, I found I understood the choices she would make beyond the page. Not just what kind of cereal she would eat or what magazines would arrive in her mail—the kinds of attributes we, as writers, are told to consider when "fleshing out" characters—but how she would live past the world I had created. How she would continue.

I offer this moment to illustrate the power of characters. If you create strong and vibrant characters, they will not be constrained by what you say about them on the page. They will become living presences in your reader's imagination and be free to wander in those wide grassy fields. Regardless of whether you are creating characters from people in your life or characters from people in your head, you have the opportunity (I would say responsibility even) to birth new beings and new versions of beings who can help us understand what it means to make our way as humans.

Dinty W. Moore, a writer I have long admired, suggests in *The Truth of the Matter* that writers create characters in three ways: description, action, and dialogue. I find his distinctions useful because they help us understand how characters are *made*—even if they are based on real human beings. While you might be lucky enough to have a character spring up, like Athena, fully formed in your head or a sibling who's as unusual as a jackalope, you still have to build that character word by word for the reader. No matter how vivid your father is in your life or the wizard is in your head, they only become real to the reader when you put the right words in the right order.

Moore begins with physical description not because it is the most compelling means for making characters but because it is the one writers often rely on—and to their detriment. Humans are visual creatures—and we tend to believe what we see with our eyes—so it makes sense that a writer would reach for physical description first. And physical detail, in and of itself, is not bad (remember the bat and the jumper cables), but we often fail to use physical detail well when creating characters. We provide the "driver license" description: medium height and brown hair. Hazel eyes. Such details tell us nothing about a person's character. Hair color rarely reveals. Instead, we want to think about specific, physical details that cement the character in our reader's head—so the reader knows exactly who we are talking about. In *Writing Fiction*, Janet Burroway gives us this description from a Margaret Atwood novel: "Mrs. Withers, the dietician, marched in through the back door, drew up, and scanned the room. She wore her usual Betty Grable hairdo and open-toed pumps, and her shoulders had an aura of shoulder pads even in a sleeveless dress."

I'm not sure about you, but for me the idea of a woman who appears to wear shoulder pads even when her shoulders are bare tells me everything I need to know about Mrs. Withers. She is not to be messed with. She is all fierce determination, no nonsense, and militaristic. I will not be crying on her shoulder. Atwood conjures Mrs. Withers by choosing the exact right physical details. When well chosen, you need only one or two. Yards and yards of lines about hair color and blue eyes will never come close to delivering what shoulder-padded bare shoulders will.

You want to choose well here. What are the specific physical details that will convey everything about a character? It's good to practice first with people in your own life. Your mother, for example. Can you choose one specific physical detail that would tell a reader exactly the kind of person your mother is? Actually try this. Write it down. One physical description. And stay far away from hair. Think about her dress. That will get you closer. Think about accessories. If I were to focus on a physical detail about my mother, I would say that she always wears matching jewelry even when dressed in jeans and a T-shirt. Try it with your own mother.

The second way we can build characters, Moore tells us, is through their actions—how they move in the world. How they hold their bodies. How they sit or stand or stir oatmeal. If we want our characters to feel three-dimensional to our reader, then they need to be three-dimensional on the page—meaning they have to be embodied beings rather than flat like a stick figure. Sometimes an action is part of a plot—one character hits another—but there is an entire canon of actions that are much more subtle and related less to cause and effect and more to how this person does or does not take up space. Maybe your character sits at the edge of the chair because they are always leaving and never staying; maybe your character wraps their arms around their bellies to hide their wounds; maybe your character refuses to pick up his dog's poop (inaction as action); maybe your character rubs their feet together every night to soothe themselves to sleep. Characters act in the world. They change the energy in the room when they enter. They bruise and they get bruised. They feel at home in their bodies or their bodies become the crime scene. Whether your characters begin in your head or in your past, when they arrive on the page, they arrive in their bodies. You want to show your reader who they are by how they move.

Return to your mothers. What is the single action you could offer that would help a reader understand exactly who your mother is? Write it down. If I were asked, I would tell you that my mother rarely takes her feet from the ground when sitting. She doesn't draw them beneath her on the couch. She doesn't place them on the coffee table. As she was taught, she never shows her soles.

Finally, and most powerfully, characters reveal themselves through their dialogue. Moore tells us that how our characters speak will say more about who they are than any other form of characterization. In the next section, we will look at the specifics of dialogue more closely, but here I just want to consider why a character's speech is so revealing—more so than their physical description or their actions. The answer lies in the way a reader receives information as they read. Physical detail and action are features that are filtered by the writer. The writer is choosing what details to share and what actions to highlight. Even though that is true for dialogue as well—the writer chooses what the character will say—the reader *experiences* dialogue as direct evidence of the character. Dialogue arrives unfiltered. This is a really important distinction: even though dialogue is equally shaped and selected by the writer, it is experienced by the reader as coming directly from the character. It feels more true. As we will see in the next chapter, dialogue creates texture and variety and physical breathing space on the page, but its brilliance comes in the way it functions as a direct pipeline to the character. It arrives as fact. Given the way it conjures truth, you can see, then, why dialogue is the strongest form of characterization.

Try it. Return to your mother. What is the one thing she might say that would tell a reader exactly who she is? If I were to return to my mother, I would offer, "You're not sick."

Description, action, and dialogue: three ways to create characters. And we rely on all three. Dialogue will be the most compelling, so lean harder in that direction, but the other two have their place. One final note that is almost too cliché to even mention, but, like all cliché, is born from truth: no reader, over the age of eight, will believe a character who is uniformly good or uniformly bad. We have spent too many years on the planet to fall for that. Honestly, we won't even grant nonhuman characters such one-dimensionality even if they are the good wizard. It's an insult to your reader to offer them either a saint or a devil for a character. In my introductory nonfiction classes, I forbid what I call "dead grandmother essays," a subgenre of essay that is doomed, almost completely, from the start. The dead grandmother is too easily sainted, too easily made wise without earning any of her wisdom, and she bakes too many muffins. I understand why my twenty-something-year-old students want to write about their dead grandmothers. For many, it is their first experience with death. But I make those grandmothers off limits as characters and topics—not because I am mean but because I know the pitfalls too well. Whether the characters come from your life or your mind or a combination of both, they can only take birth on the page if they, like all of us, have been marked by the world. In the same vein, they, like all of us, must always have the possibility of redemption. We all fail; we all rise. So, too, must those who wander our stories.

Finally, it is important to realize, especially for those of us writing nonfiction, that sacred spaces exist in our lives—these are the real people we are unwilling to trouble on the page. For example, I rarely write directly about my husband, Michael, or at least not in extended ways. I know that I am unwilling to name his warts. He has them. I assure you. But because he remains sacred to me, because I won't complicate him for the reader, I don't really write about him. I must recognize just who in my life is off limits—*not* because I am censoring myself or am afraid to write about them but because I am not ready to complicate them. Know and respect what is sacred to you. Save what is sacred for your heart and not your art. The page always requires a writer to risk. You are in charge of when and how to take those risks.

30

Whose Line Is It?

When I chose to pursue a doctorate, creative PhD programs did not exist, or, if they did, they were so few in number, I had never heard of them. Even if I had, I am not sure at the age of twenty-five and newly divorced, I would have chosen to follow fiction. That would have felt too risky to me, and I was already scrubbing hard at the word failure that I imagined stamped across my forehead. So I chose to study composition and rhetoric—or maybe, and I like to think this, composition and rhetoric chose me: that the universe knew that I needed to begin my life as a creative writer by learning how writing worked and how to teach it. I have always been grateful that I arrived at art through craft. Composition and rhetoric, as a field, taught me to value the labor of writing, to keep my head down, feet on the ground, and see writing as a way of knowing rather than an end in itself.

Maybe having arrived late to orientation or maybe not knowing the right people or maybe just being the new kid on the block, my first semester at Michigan I was assigned a 7:30 a.m. class of first-year composition that met in a dilapidated brick building half a mile off campus. The time slot alone should have sunk me, not to mention the long walk in the increasingly colder fall mornings, but I thrived in that class, looked forward to the time with my students, spent hours responding to their work. That semester, alone in a new place, still stinging from my divorce, and far from the Hawaiian sun, should have been terrible, but I remember strong coffee and cold mornings and sitting in a circle with my students talking about their writing. I remember warmth.

Even though grading rubrics were pretty much unheard of at the university level at that time, I had just come from teaching middle school and believed that rubrics helped make visible what was so often invisible: the attributes of "good" writing. Students in first-year composition at the University of Michigan were asked to write argumentative essays—traditional academic writing that begins with a clear thesis and then proceeds to argue for that thesis through the use of textual evidence. Whether they were writing about the death penalty or the superiority of bagels to doughnuts, I found that my students struggled to find the right kind of evidence to support their thesis statements. Too often, their evidence seemed to float like lonely buoys in their essays, tethered to nothing and useful to no one. In an effort to make visible the attributes of strong evidence, I created a rubric that rewarded evidence that was both directed and discerning—directed in that each piece of evidence was relevant to the point being made and discerning in that it was well chosen, that it appeared to be pulled from the heap of possible pieces of evidence by a writer with a clear understanding of what was valuable.

Dialogue is evidence.

Hence, dialogue needs to be directed and discerning.

Dialogue is the only opportunity for a reader to access information that comes straight from the characters. All the rest of the information in an essay or a story (setting, scene, significant detail, metaphor, etc.) is filtered by the writer. Dialogue feels, to the reader, unfiltered. It's, of course, not, but it *feels* that way. Readers welcome dialogue because those are the moments where the reader makes their own decisions about the characters, whether they are to be trusted, whether they are good, whether they are likable. Nothing stands in the way of the reader and what the characters are saying. If scenes unfold in real time, then the dialogue in those scenes are moments where the characters whisper directly into the reader's ears. It is intimate, close.

You want to choose your dialogue well. Just as we arrive in the scene as close as possible to the climax of the scene, we arrive in dialogue as close as possible to the evidence the dialogue is going to provide. The reader expects to be shown something in a scene—otherwise why are we in a scene—and they most often look to the dialogue for the place where the evidence will be revealed. Start close to the climax with your dialogue. Don't ask the reader to wade through undirected and undiscerned tracts of conversation. Don't ask the reader to try and figure out why they are there. The reader should know why they have arrived and then, to some degree, be surprised by what they learn; they should leave both the scene and the dialogue within the scene with a more complicated understanding of the story or the essay.

Beyond its central role at providing direct evidence to the reader, dialogue creates texture on the page. Remember that each character will be revealed most clearly by what they say, so every time they speak, it will add a new voice to the writing. A different pitch or tone. Without dialogue, we only have the voice of the narrator—not an impossible approach but a challenging one. A piece without dialogue can feel flat to the reader, like they are trapped in a room alone with only one version of reality to consider. Dialogue adds nuance, perspective, alternatives, and waves. Because dialogue is traditionally punctuated by indenting every time a new character speaks, dialogue also creates physical breathing space on the page. The reader will experience a spaciousness when they arrive at dialogue, even if the dialogue itself is tense or terse. Readers welcome that breath.

Lastly, because dialogue must always be discerning (wheat not chaff), it is not the place to dump information. Use summary to give readers background information, or, better yet, find a way to convey needed information through scenic detail. When a character speaks, a reader listens. They value what is being said. Dialogue is not the place for a character to tell a reader how many siblings they have or how long they have lived in Indiana or what they ate for breakfast. Unless that information is going to change the direction of the plot or complicate the central question, then you don't want it in your dialogue.

Your characters will not speak very often. Choose your dialogue like you would choose a parachute, with care, with intention, with an understanding of the stakes. As the writer, you are in charge of choosing the best possible dialogue, and then the reader is in charge of deciding what that dialogue means for them. Think about your own reading experience. Say, you have to read a novel for a class and you haven't given yourself enough time to finish it. You might look for a summary online, but you might also start to skim. And what will you be looking for as you skim? My guess would be dialogue. Because you know that dialogue is the place where important things are happening.

Below is a section of dialogue from a flash essay by Ira Sukrungruang entitled "To Disappear & To Find." In it, the author and his toddler son are driving through an empty Ohio landscape on a route they take every day to school. They pass a lone tree in a field and his son speaks.

"Daddy, turn around and look at the tree."

"I can't."

"Sure, you can."

"Daddy has to keep both hands on the wheel and his eyes on the road."

"No, you don't."

"Yes, I do." We go back and forth between my yeses and his noes. "If Daddy takes his eyes off the road we can get into an accident."

"What's an accident?"

"It's when we lose control of the car and hit something."

"Like a tree?"

I nod.

"But there're no trees." My son points to the outside flat blurring by.

"Not in Ohio."

"Daddy, what happens in an accident?"

"Sometimes people get hurt."

"What happens when people get hurt?"

"Remember when you scrapped your knee? It's like that but worse."

"What worse?"

"Like you can—" I don't finish the sentence. I don't want to tell my son you can hurt so bad you die. I don't want to explain the word "die." Or dying. Or death. Even if it's foremost on my mind. Even when many have passed recently—family, friends, and teachers. The moment I knew my son was coming into the world, I flashed ahead—he only a worm in his mother's womb—to a tomorrow where I'm dead, and fearing I hadn't prepared him for this brutal life.

Or a life without me.

The essay continues, almost entirely in dialogue. Dialogue, like the above, that is filled with the inexplicability of death—words that cannot name the truth. And the lines are all fairly short, which is ironic given the essay's deeper subject: the reality of this often brutal life. Sukrungruang's responses to his son arrive thin and fragile, just like his own existence. Because it is nonfiction, we also read the essay within its historical context, a year into the pandemic. Many are disappearing at the same moment that many continue to appear. The dialogue here says more by saying less with neither writer or reader able to articulate the pain of loss but both feeling it nonetheless. All by allowing the characters to speak.

31

What to Bring to Show and Tell

When I was eight, in the months after I resumed attending second grade for the entire day, I brought my favorite record album to school for Show and Tell. We had been told to choose something precious to share with our classmates and, in groups of three, assigned specific dates. The teacher said we could share anything we wanted as long as it fit in a paper bag and wasn't alive. At those stipulations, many of my classmates whined in complaint, but my family had no pets since we moved so often; it would never have occurred to me to bring an animal. Besides, I knew immediately what I wanted to share.

Maybe because it was near the holiday season, I chose to bring my Rudolph the Red-Nosed Reindeer record to school, the one I listened to every night while falling asleep, the voice of Burl Ives as familiar as the image of Rudolph flying across the cover. To protect the record, I placed it behind my back when I took my seat on the school bus. For the entire ride up and down the hills of northern Virginia, oak limbs bare and acorns crunching beneath bus tires, I pressed my back against the vinyl. I could feel its stiff presence the entire time. But, in the hum and hurry of arriving at school, elementary kids pouring from doors like rivers, I forgot the record on the bus. When I realized what had happened, I begged the teacher to let me go to the office and see if I could call the bus driver; the teacher would not relent. By then, they would not have allowed me to leave the room unless I could point to blood.

During Show and Tell that day, my heart hammered in my chest. I was sure that the record was lost and, with it, the story, heard every night, reassuring in its stable repeatability. Other kids shared books and action figures and planes built from plastic parts and glue, while I sat with my arms crossed and mourned the loss of something else in my life. That afternoon, the bus driver returned the record to me amid a cacophony of voices claiming the record as their own. Once I had the album safely in my hands, I slid the record from its cover and saw the vinyl cracked in two.

No doubt you have heard the writerly advice "show don't tell." And perhaps you, too, can remember moments from your elementary days when you had the opportunity to share something you loved with your classmates. I think it useful to recall the fact that you had the chance to both show *and* tell. There you are, standing at the front of the room, addressing your peers, model airplane in hand. We ought to be wary of any writing advice that insists on binaries: this not that. Art is not calculus. Nothing is simply right or wrong. One of my favorite yoga teachers, Bernie Clark, says, "Never is never right and always is always wrong." We want to embrace the "and" of show and tell.

Much of what we have been considering—scenes, characters, dialogue—are the very craft elements a writer uses to *show* a reader what is happening in a story or a poem or an essay. If you think back to the first part of this book, we began with the idea that an artist's entire pursuit is aimed at externalizing something experienced or felt or known on the incoherent, intangible, and unmanifest inside. Writing is an attempt to externalize the internal. I think about the final lines of one of Georgia O'Keeffe's letters when she is writing to Alfred Stieglitz about her early abstractions in charcoal: "I make them—just to express myself—things I feel and want to say—haven't words for—You probably know without my saying it—that I ask because I wonder if I got over to anyone what I want to say." We, as writers, as artists, are always wondering if we "got over to anyone" what we want to say. In the literary arts, showing is the place we begin in our attempt to externalize. We rely on images, significant details, complex characters, and well-chosen scenes. "Can you see this?" we ask our real or imagined readers. Do you understand? Have I put enough of the right words in the right order to convey what lives inside of me so that it can start to live inside of you?

Such an act—so magical, so alchemical, not only a complete transformation of something inchoate inside you into a manifest form, into language, but also a transference of those words into the lived experience of another being—such an act requires that we, as writers, show as much as possible. Reveal. Describe. Illumine. We will never fully succeed. What lives inside of me can never live entirely inside of you. But we try to "get over to anyone," even if we know we will fail. There is a line from the *Laṅkāvatāra Sutra* that speaks to this: "Just as a fool, on seeing a moon-pointing finger, looks at the finger but not the moon, so one who is attached to words does not see the Real." Words only point, as does paint or clay. The word "moon" is not the moon itself. But words name the moon, birth the moon into shared existence. When we use language to show—through image, metaphor, significant detail, concrete nouns, strong verbs, well-chosen scenes, complex characters, precise dialogue—the reader begins to see our version of the moon. In effect, writer and reader stand together and observe what the words are pointing to. The moons they see will never be the same, but, the more a writer can show the reader what their moon looks like, the closer the two images of moon grow.

In our writing, we also have the option of telling, and I am going to suggest two ways in which telling becomes as powerful as showing. The first is through interiority, something fiction writers are especially good at. Interiority occurs when a reader is allowed inside the mind of a character. The reader learns what a character thinks or believes. Done poorly, it can feel as if the writer doesn't know how to show us what the character feels (through action and direct dialogue) so they are taking a shortcut and telling us. That is the danger of telling and why language arts teachers spend so much energy making sure a writer never tells. Just as novice writers can rely on summary too much because creating scenes is difficult, they can rely on telling us what the character is thinking because it is easier than showing. They hope they can get away with it, but they can't. Interiority does not take the place of character development but rather adds another layer.

Here is the opening of the third chapter of Toni Morrison's novel *Paradise*: "Either the pavement was burning or she had sapphires hidden in her shoes. K.D., who had never seen a woman mince or switch like that, believed it was the walk that caused all the trouble." We are inside K.D.'s head, learning how he sees the world. He blames Gigi, the woman stepping from the bus, for what comes to pass in the small town of Mercy. This is not the narrator's voice. Here is that voice: "If ever there came a morning when mercy and simple good fortune took to their heels and fled, grace alone might have to do. But from where would it come and how fast? In that holy hollow between sighting and following through, could grace slip through it all?" Nor is K.D. talking with other characters. It's a pipeline right into K.D.'s head. Now, if we spent all of our time, as readers, inside K.D.'s head, we might grow tired (though there are entire novels that are stream of consciousness novels where we never leave a character's head). We are grateful for the peek into K.D.'s head and then happy to watch K.D. interact with the other characters, especially knowing what we know about how he sees Gigi. Telling adds; it doesn't take away.

There is a second, more political reason to make sure we, as writers, have access to both showing and telling. As we saw a few chapters ago, musing and reflection are a kind of telling and are an important aspect of memoir in particular. Recently, writers have pointed to the fact that the maxim "show don't tell" can work to reinscribe trauma, particularly physical and sexual abuse. A survivor who was told by their abuser to never tell is faced with a serious challenge when a teacher insists they "show don't tell." As Sonya Huber argues in "The Three Words That Almost Ruined Me as a Writer," such advice "repeats the abuse [students] will have endured along with its highest commandment: secrecy." In addition, the insistence on showing alone puts all the emphasis on scene and action and can make a writer feel that their story or essay or poem must always be dramatic and extraordinary. But some stories, stories from the margins in particular, are lost when we forsake telling for showing. As Huber continues, "We know that if we reduce ourselves to actions and surface details—what can be seen—many of us will disappear."

Show *and* tell. There's a reason our elementary school teachers had us both bring an object to share and tell the class about it. We need both. Always is always wrong and never is never right.

32

What Piano?

I like to think of writing as alchemy. Later, I will describe in more detail how writing requires both involution and evolution and how an understanding of alchemy can help us think about our work. I would add here that yoga is alchemical as well—maybe not the yoga that people do in the gym while the barbells crash overhead, but rather the deeper dimensions of yoga where the body becomes the pathway to liberation. Actually, alchemy surrounds us: morning becomes afternoon; winter becomes spring; a banana becomes our body; oxygen transforms into carbon dioxide with every breath. If alchemy is simply transformation, then our world is entirely alchemical, for nothing, not even the mountains, escapes change. But any alchemist will tell you that transformation on its own is not alchemy. An alchemist follows the motto: *labora et ora*. Work and prayer. Alchemy, like yoga and writing, requires not just practice but also intention. You must bring your entire being into the lab; otherwise, you are just cooking dinner.

Writing reveals its alchemical nature at the level of the word. Words take us down the alchemical ladder, moving from what is unknown or inchoate into something that is more fixed, less fluid. Language allows us to evolve from what Audre Lorde describes as "the nameless and formless about to be birthed, but already felt" into, say, the word "table." A table, most of us will agree, has four legs and a top. When I say the word "table," we will all have varying images of a table in our heads but most all of them will have four legs and a surface. There is, of course, no law that dictates such a structure need be called a "table." It could be called a "wampus." But English speakers have agreed to name that structure "table." When we name something, it becomes fixed. It loses fluidity. Whatever its table-like nature was before we seized it and named it "table" is hard to recover. Rarely, if ever, do we consider its tableness. We honestly would have trouble seeing the tableness of a table without envisioning an actual table. Try it. Try and *feel* the tableness of a table without picturing a table. Feel table without seeing a table in your head or thinking the word "table."

Hard to do. Yet, that is exactly how an alchemist widens their perception so that they can more freely ascend up and down the alchemical ladder. It's a good practice for a writer because, as writers, we have a lot of faith in words. We might assume that the words we put down on the page are the very same words that our readers will pick up and carry. And they can't be. My table is not your table even if we all agree "table" means a structure with four legs and a top. Westerners in particular—so often linear thinkers who tend to prize rationality above intuition—have trouble not believing the text. Look, we say, it says so right there, but the "there" is not really there. Nothing exists, of substance, beneath the word "table." Under table or within table or below table is tableness. And tableness, as we just saw, is pretty hard to experience.

An alchemist sees behind or beneath or below words. They try to isolate the subtle qualities, elemental qualities, of a substance. When an alchemist "turns" lead into gold, they are not actually turning lead into gold but rather they are exalting the elements of lead, purifying them, to their most subtle nature, their divinity let's say, and that is the gold.

Language works, for the most part, as an evolute. Words are the solidified results of subtle nature—Lordes' "nameless and formless about to be birthed"—taking birth, shape, form. An alchemist might call words the gross or the *prima materia*. The gross is made heavy by the fact that it has become so mixed up, polluted even, by the manifest world. All divinity, all gold, is hidden, gone. The word "table" has lost its tableness. Table becomes hard, fixed, determined, and not all that interesting.

But, and here is the joy, language can move up the alchemical ladder and involute—return a substance to its less fixed, more divine form. And one way to do this is through metaphor. Metaphors are the single most magical element of our language. They take a word that is frozen and determined and exalt the word to a higher state, one less fixed, more free, and closer to its nature of being.

When Toni Morrison, alchemist second to none, tells the reader that her character has opened "a menu of regret" she begins the alchemical process. Menu is concrete and fixed. We will all see our version of menu when we read the word (mine is tan colored). But Morrison latches menu to regret (a less fixed noun, more abstract, but still commonly held). As readers, we bring together menu and regret and the combination of the two transforms into a substance that is not so easily defined. Menu of regret is so much more expansive and fluid than a simple menu or an empty abstraction like regret. Loss comes in whole courses—appetizers when we are younger and then main dishes. You might order sides of regret as well. Or those sides might come with the main meal. No substitutions allowed. We categorize regret, try and make it nice and neat, but the menu gets bent and stained over the years; there are crossouts, price changes, and new suppliers. My menu of regret is heavy and formal. Stiff. Items are being added all the time. I carry my menu of regret with me always, can open it like I might the weather app. Morrison forged my menu for me the first time I read her spell.

That is metaphor. The concrete and the abstract are joined and something more profound and more fluid gets distilled. A menu of regret conjures neither menu nor regret but something else entirely, something less seen and more felt. We have moved upward—leaving the concrete and working to return to the very nature, the very essence of our humanity.

Metaphor—a subset of figurative language that includes the equally magical figures of imagery as well as paradox, metonymy, simile, and so on—must arise organically from the work. You don't import imagery into your writing; imagery distills from the work itself. Sometimes when writers reach for metaphor, they look outside of their story or poem and seize an image that has no relation to what they are making. For example, a character lies beneath the chassis of a car, working on an engine, hands covered in grease. From the garage door, unwilling to leave the warmth of the house, their mother screams at them for not taking the garbage to the curb. Worthless, the mother calls the child, stupid as well. But when the character begins to bang the crescent wrench against a bolt that won't turn, the writer compares their efforts to banging the keys of the piano.

What?! The reader asks. Piano? Where did the piano come from? The reader pokes their head up from the dream; the spell evaporates.

What if, instead, the writer stays with the character beneath the belly of the car, doesn't reach outside the scene for a piano, but, instead, the character hammers the bolt like a miner in a vein who has lost their way back to the surface. Better. Maybe not perfect but better. Mines are dark and claustrophobic. They are cold, unmapped, tight. And you can die beneath the earth without any air. Pianos don't often suffocate.

I would argue that more magic is happening when the character is likened to a miner caught beneath the weight of their mother's anger than when a piano takes the stage, and that's because the underside of a car conjures a cave more readily than a musical instrument. More to the point, both the physical setting and the abstract quality of the mother's anger become transmuted when they are brought together. The underside of the car and her anger become more fluid, dynamic, and expansive.

Try it. Return to the character exercises from a few chapters back—the ones where you turned your mother into a character by isolating a physical detail, a turn of phrase, and an action. Put that character into a scene, an ordinary room in the house. Have her act and speak and move within that room. She can be alone or with others. Fiction or nonfiction. Allow yourself a single metaphor or simile. Think about the general emotion of the moment, the energy in the room. And pay attention to those tables, those lamps, the rug on the floor. We alchemize the ordinary back to the divine. Here is my fictional attempt:

My mother sits in the darkness at 2:00 a.m. Her husband left the house hours ago to walk the beach of their vacation rental somewhere on the Delaware coast. Or maybe to find a liquor store. Or maybe just to drive. The living room windows are closed, so she can only imagine the sound of surf. In the silence, the cooling coils of the refrigerator buzz to life right at the moment she drops her slingback heels to the floor like pelts. The blanket she finds on the back of the armchair cannot reach her feet.

33

The Body Is Your Swing

In *My Grandmother's Hands: Racialized Trauma and the Pathway to Mending Our Hearts and Bodies*, Resmaa Menakem explores the way trauma is stored in the body. We tend to think of trauma as something that happens to us, but really trauma is something that dis-members us, disembodies us, casts us from our only homes. White-body supremacy, Menakem tells us, has traumatized all bodies. As with patriarchy and capitalism, no one escapes unharmed by inequality. Black bodies and Brown bodies and Red bodies, of course, have been traumatized the most by White-body supremacy, but White bodies need also to understand how they have been dis-membered by their unacknowledged and unearned privilege. As Menakem writes, "trauma always happens *in the body*," so you cannot look to the rational brain to unlearn racist behavior or recover from racist abuse. We can't *think* our ways out of racism. Instead, we must turn to our bodies as sources for re-membering who we are and how we want to live in this world.

    I bring up Menakem's work here because he takes us to somatic, or bodily, experience as not just *a* way to heal ourselves but as *the* only way. And not just healing from White-body supremacy. We must heal from all the ways in which the world breaks us open. All of us are marked. Some more visibly than others. All of us are scarred and wounded, beginning with the initial wound that comes from entering the world from a space where all your needs were met to one in which you learn hunger. All of us, then, must be returned to our bodies.

    We can add somatic movement to the breath to keep us in our bodies, especially if we are having trouble focusing on the breath or we are experiencing greater levels of anxiety. Repetitive, rhythmic motions help activate the vagus nerve, the soul nerve, and the part of our nervous system that calms us. If you are like me, you might already be engaging in some of these soothing techniques, but you may not have named them as healing or even as a technique. It's just what your body does. For example, long before I understood the science behind the movements, I would rock and sway.

Often when seated. It just felt good in my body to move side to side. I am also someone who has hummed my entire life—when driving, or washing dishes, or waiting for the dentist—just under my breath, lips vibrating quietly. Most often, I did both at the same time, but I wouldn't have been able to tell you that I was caring for myself. I just hummed and swayed, swayed and hummed. There is a deep down biological reason for the fact that we rock babies in our arms and sing to them. *Both* parent and child are calmed by the action. Since we have climbed out of both heart and body to take up residence in our hard-edged, judgmental, dualistic minds, we have to re-member our way back to our only homes. We have to feel, physically feel, our bodies again.

Below, I list several somatic practices that you can add to your breath work—or actually do any time of the day—that return you to your body, quiet your mind, and allow you to be entirely present for your life and your art. As you engage in these practices, keep in mind the words of Bonnie Bainbridge Cohen: "The mind is like the wind and the body is like the sand; if you want to know how the wind is blowing, you can look at the sand." Somatic practices keep us focused on the sand.

One somatic technique to try is tapping. While much has been written on Emotional Freedom Technique, or EFT, I arrived at tapping through my research on acupressure points and Traditional Chinese Medicine. Tapping is something I incorporate into my yoga classes as well as my writing classes. At the most basic level, tapping reminds us that we are not our thoughts; we are a body. A more nuanced discussion of tapping would include a study of how energy moves through the subtle body to arrive at meridian points. Acupressure, or pressure on these points, helps to balance the physical and energetic bodies, a kind of acupuncture but without the needles. I only want to provide the most simple tapping exercise here and the one I use most often. If you enjoy the practice, then I would encourage you to read and explore more.

Begin with your four- and six-count breath. Establish stillness in your body. Then begin by lightly tapping your temples. It doesn't matter if you use one or two fingers, nor does it matter which fingers you use, first, second, both. Tap lightly at both temples with your eyes closed. After a few moments, travel down to the space just beneath your eyes and tap there. Travel back up around the eyes and maybe pause at the temples again before moving up along the brow line to the edge of the brow. Tap there. Then continue back down around the eye and tap again under the eyes. Perhaps move to the inside edge of the nose and then back to the temples. You can decide to follow the cheekbones out and tap at the hinge of the jaw. Linger. Maybe now follow the hinge back and tap just below the ears. Follow the chin line and tap at the center of the chin below the bottom lip (maybe just one hand for that). Then retrace your steps. Think of yourself as outlining your face or walking a path around your face, not unlike how practitioners in India circumambulate a temple three times before entering to pray. Walk your face like you would a secret garden or a woodsy trail. Trace your face the way your mother may have, or wished she did, when you couldn't fall asleep or were sick. Pause wherever it feels good to pause and linger for as long as it feels good to remain. Maybe you never move from the first place.

Other places to tap would be right at the sternum, with one hand, just above the heart center. The sound is hollow there. You can move from that space to the two acupressure points that exist just below the divot in your collarbones right above each breast. You can also decide not to tap but to lightly press these places. Make small circles. Sometimes these spots will feel slightly painful or a bit raw. That's actually a good thing. In TCM, that would indicate blocked energy or some lodged sorrow. Applying pressure will release some of that blocked energy. While there are exact acupressure points on your body, you do not need to know where they are. The point is the tapping. Think of it as lightly knocking at the door of a house that you own but have somehow lost the key for. Tap with love. Tap with care. You are asking to return to yourself. When you are done tracing your face or your heart, then sit for a minute and just breathe. Feel that.

A second option for somatic experience is to simply sway as you breathe. Seated with crossed legs or in a chair works best for this. Again, find stillness first. Then close your eyes and just let your body sway side to side or forward and back. There is no right or wrong. Swaying is the point. Big sways, little sways, just the body, just the head, both head and body, it doesn't matter. The image I always conjure in this practice, because the ocean is so central to my life, is the sway of seaweed on the ocean floor. It moves with the breath of the ocean, carried by an unseen current. You may be more familiar with the sway of a giant tree in a gentle wind, limbs lifting and releasing, the tree giving shape to the invisible force of air. Or perhaps you think of prairie grass. Or maybe a swing unclaimed by a child, moving on its own. Sway from your body, not from your mind. Rock yourself the way your parents once rocked you or you once rocked your child or your dog or your favorite stuffed animal. Sway and breathe, breathe and sway. After a few minutes, return to stillness. Let the sway continue long past when the body halts.

Lastly, hum. Humming is the most portable of these practices, for you can hum a tune as you shower or water the flowers, pick up dog poop, take the car through the carwash. And you can hum anything from "Amazing Grace" to "Sweet Child o' Mine" or a tune all your own. Humming alone will certainly calm you. But you can also deepen that practice with more intention. There is a specific yoga breath practice called *bhramari* or bee's breath. This *prāṇāyāma* is one of the oldest recorded yoga practices that we know of and is found in the *Hatha Yoga Pradīpika*, a fifteenth-century text by Swami Svātmārāma. In the simplest form of this practice, you simply inhale through your nose for the count of four and then, when you exhale, you exhale a hum or buzz, like a bee. It helps to seal your lips on exhalation.

Inhale again and then exhale and hum. To deepen the somatic experience, you can close your eyes and plug your ears with your fingers. The hum will vibrate through your entire body. Remain with the bee breath for several minutes and then pause. Place your hands in your lap. Feel the way your body continues to hum long after you have stopped. It's like your body is calling to you: remember me. The *Hatha Yoga Pradīpika* says of this breath, "Thus a certain bliss and delight are born in the minds of good yogis from doing *bhramari*." Bliss and delight.

34

Creating Our Own Obstacles

Hanuman is a beloved god in India. A divine personality belonging to the Vanara community, Hanuman is known as the leaper of obstacles as well as the god of compassion and the perfect devotee. His story can be found alongside the story of Rama and Sita in the mighty Indian epic the *Ramayana*, a tale that spans some 700 pages and recounts the fourteen years that Rama, an incarnation of the god Vishnu, spent wandering the forest in exile. At the center of the story lies the demon Ravana's decision to steal Sita, Rama's dutiful and beautiful wife, and take her to Lanka, where he locks her away in a garden. To make a very, very long story short, Hanuman finds Sita in Lanka and ultimately brings her home to Rama. The island Lanka sits off the southern coast of India. No one in Rama's service, none of the other warriors or monkeys, can make the leap from the tip of India to the island. Only Hanuman can. But, and here is one of my favorite parts of the story, Hanuman does not remember that Vayu, the god of the wind, is his father and that he is a demigod. He does not recall that he is divine. As a child, he leaped too high into the sky and threatened the god Indra. For that action, Hanuman was cursed to never remember his divinity.

When he stands, or actually kneels in many versions, at the tip of the Indian subcontinent and prepares for what seems impossible, he prays for something that he already has. Then he raises his gaze and makes the jump.

I could write forever about Hanuman. Hanuman lives everywhere in India, as ubiquitous as Ganesha. Unlike Shiva, who can be quick to anger, or Kali, with her blood-soaked tongue, Hanuman is easy to love for he so clearly mimics our own story: we are all born full and perfect and then we forget.

Our journey in this life is to remember our wholeness and goodness. It is the reaching, craving, and wanting in our lives that leads to most of our suffering.

"This is what is," the universe says.

And then we respond, "Okay, but what I'd really like is a ham sandwich, or a new job, shinier hair, more hair, less fat, a fast car."

"This is what is," says the universe again.

And rather than say, okay, yes, this is what is, rather than accept what is unfolding right now in front of us, we protest that what we are being offered is uncomfortable or unattractive or just the wrong color. In yoga, this wanting/craving is termed *rāga* and the pushing away/aversion is called *dveṣa*. Together, and quite simply, *rāga* and *dveṣa* create our unhappiness.

What is *is* what is. To act in any other way is pure madness. Yet, we do it all day long.

I am not saying we can't work to change our lives, but we can only enact change when we first accept where we are. Clarity must precede hope.

Myths of all sorts—from Ancient Greek to Indian to those passed down by indigenous peoples—are profound sites for wisdom when we understand that we play every role in the story. Every character in every myth is an aspect of ourselves. We are the demon who simply wants to take what is pretty. We are the king who has been cast from home. We are the one who can leap across any distance. And the one who forgets that this is true. When we fail to realize that we already have everything that we need, and we begin to think that if we had more or less of something then we would be just fine, we create our own obstacles. The leap becomes impossible, so we do nothing. Or we scroll our phone. Or eat some chocolate.

Hanuman's leap is a long way for me to arrive at my central point in this chapter, which is that I don't believe in writer's block. I believe that writers think they are blocked and can't write, but I think that block is created by us. Just like we create so many obstacles to our own happiness. I am not saying that we don't face real difficulty, real loss, real suffering. Nor am I saying that we just need to keep our chin up and smile. Rather, in every moment we have what we need to do what we need to do. We just have to remember.

Writers say they are blocked for all sorts of reasons—they can't figure out what happens next in their story; they haven't done the research that they need to do; their writing sucks; their poem sucks; they suck. And I don't doubt for a second that when a writer tells me that they are stuck that they don't feel stuck. They do. But they also have the capacity to leap. They just need to remember that they are born to write, that they have all that they need, and that they are, indeed, whole. Nothing is missing. Nothing is wanting. We live in a culture that constantly suggests we lack, and it's easy to see why we start to believe it. But Vayu is our father. Wind whistles in our bones. When we think we are stuck and can no longer write, we can find our feet again by doing any of the following:

- Engage in more low-stakes writing. I have yet to hear someone tell me that they are stuck in their writer's notebook. For them, the writing notebook isn't a possible place to *be* stuck. Why? Because nothing specific is supposed to be happening in the writer's notebook. Anything is fine. It's when they move to their laptop or to the "page" that somehow now something else is supposed to be happening and they feel incapable of making that something else happen. Writer's block only happens, in my experience, with high-stakes writing. Lower your stakes. Return to your notebook. Remember: there is nowhere to go. We are not writing to publish or author or win the Pulitzer. We are writing because we have to write. If all writing is knowing, there is no way to fail.

- On a more literal level, there are many craft exercises you can do when you feel stuck on a certain project. Have one character or speaker write a letter to another character or speaker; have one character or speaker write a diary entry or several entries; write a letter to your mother explaining your latest essay; allow the lamp or the rug or the dog to create the scene or tell the story; change from first-person narration to second or third.

- Finally, change your genre entirely. Stop working on that story. Write a poem instead—a poem that has nothing to do with your story or your characters or your life. A poem about a police officer, perhaps.

We can always find a reason not to write or get out of bed or have a difficult conversation. There are days where I walk around my house and only see what is wrong—the need for new paint, the worn carpet, the underside of the couch where the cats have pulled out the stuffing. Really, the list is endless. I can kneel at the edge of my continent and spend my days beseeching the universe to produce something else in my life. Or I can lower the stakes. Acknowledge that both of my socks match, that I am loved (at least by the cats), and that I only need to write in my notebook about how much I hate the month of January or maybe ten ways to describe the leaden skies. In the present moment, we have everything that we need. A block is only a block if we make it so. Another way to think about an obstacle is a forced opportunity that has come our way.

35

Research and Laundry

When creative nonfiction writer Philip Gerard describes the research that he completed for his book on the Civil War, he focuses on walking the hills of Gettysburg, coming to understand, in his body, in the beat of his heart, that soldiers were moving uphill when they attacked, allowing himself, for a moment, to breathe as hard as they would have. He writes of the experience, "There is no substitute for being there, for doing it—whatever 'it' is."

If your understanding of research begins and ends in front of a computer or among the library stacks, then you probably run from the idea of research and say silly things like how you don't want to be influenced by others. If you think research belongs only to the nonfiction writers, then you have given away some of your best tools. All writers conduct research, often throughout the writing process. While research does include sitting at your kitchen table with an actual book in front of you and taking notes in your notebook as you read, compiling quotations with page numbers, dates, names, significant points, it also includes a quick Google search to learn the standard fare served in a TV dinner in the late 1970s; it includes checking the national weather database to figure out how cold it would be along the Platte River in Nebraska on an early day in April before your characters step out of the car; it includes sitting in front of a library shelf where you have found a single book that looks promising and then skimming all the books on the same shelf to find books you may have missed; it includes tasting Nutella; it includes holding the diary of your great-great-great-aunt; it includes conversations with a mechanic to understand how a starter works, or conversations with a war veteran to understand a typical day in Kuwait, or conversations with your mother about the days just after your father's death when your grandmother arrived and insisted on raising you; it includes sitting under the sun in the West Desert of Utah in July and knowing its hammerfall; it includes crying in a dark room because your heart has been broken and remembering just how literal that breaking feels in your body. Honestly, there is absolutely nothing outside your experience that is not ultimately a kind of research for your work. If, fundamentally, we write to know, then our entire world becomes the field for our knowing. Paradoxically, while research has no limits, it also doesn't just happen. We have to be as intentioned in our research as we are in our breathing. And, once again, we have to do the work.

The poet Paisley Rekdal spent more than a year conducting research for her poem "West: A Translation," a poem that marks the driving of the Golden Spike in 1869 by questioning, alongside Thoreau, whose bodies the rails ride on. Before writing a line, she accumulated more than eighty pages of research notes; she read "every poem ever written about trains in America." In an effort to recover what can never be recovered—the death of 20,000 laborers whose names remain lost to history—Rekdal recorded refrains spoken in the language of those who built the railroad: Navajo, Greek, Shoshone, Polish, and Chinese. She also conducted site visits where she walked desert lands and empty towns. While those landscapes may initially appear empty, Rekdal found them full of ghosts. She writes of her field work,

> It was so amazing to be able to reach down and pick up a physical piece of history. I remember picking up this button I couldn't believe I was holding, basically a trouser button from somebody's pants. That was just there and had been there for 150 years. The sort of reminder that this is not a fantasy. This is not something in the past. In some ways it's still part of our present and we could just reach out and touch it.

To write a single poem (in full disclosure, the poem itself is epic and far from short), Rekdal conducted every kind of research possible. She did not sit in her living room and write about the triumphant moment when that last spike was driven and the east met the west in northern Utah. She stepped into mess, complication, and competing voices. She stepped out of her car and onto the ground.

It helps to think of research in two general categories and to access them both. They both have value. Gerard makes the distinction between living research and archival research, and we can learn from that division. Archival research is the research found on a computer, in the library, and in the archives. It contains both primary materials (letters, newspapers, diaries, ship manifests, and photos) and secondary materials (books, articles, and essays *about* primary materials). I believe in good old-fashioned research as a place to begin. Think of your archival work as creating a much needed context for you as a writer. Whether investigating a certain time period, event, geography, or person, archival research is what *lets you know the questions to ask*. You cannot ask good questions of yourself, your characters, your interview subjects, or the work itself unless you have steeped yourself in background. Deep dive. Let's say you want to understand how Tarot works. Sure, you can Google and find out from Wikipedia that Tarot is a pack of playing cards used for divination with ties to the occult. But until you begin deep research into Tarot, you won't understand how Tarot is medicinal.

I typically suggest that writers begin with archival research and fill notebooks with all that they find. Librarians can be really helpful as can online searches and access to a university library but also walk the stacks. Or, if you are working in Special Collections, make sure to look at associated boxes and folders. At the beginning, move wide and then deepen once you understand the questions you have. Questions always drive your research. If you ask it, then try to answer it. Writers often want to know when they have done enough archival research. One way I respond is practical: once you recognize the references being made in what you are reading and at least know of those references even if you haven't read them, you are close. Your research starts to feel less like a line and more like a circle. Less practical but more likely, you leave your archival research because you have a deadline that you need to honor. Most writers I know would research their passions for the rest of their lives—and many do.

The second kind of research is called living research and involves moving your body. Living research includes the interviews and conversations you have with experts in the area or just the people who appear as you conduct a site visit. It's really any interaction or conversation you have surrounding your subject—whether with your mother or the head of the Strategy and Policy Department at the Naval War College. These conversations can provide additional background information, specialized information, or evolve into characters in the work itself. Living research involves going to places that are important to your project and walking those hills or picking up that button. As Gerard says, there is no substitute for being there.

Whether conducting archival or living research, you want to take copious notes. You think you will remember. You won't. Your writer's notebook will come in handy here. I dedicate entire notebooks to certain projects and fill them with journal entries as well as my research notes. The fiction writer Amor Towles has an office brimming with notebooks of research for possible novels. Of his research, he says,

> There's a multi-year design phase when an idea has grabbed my attention. I'm thinking about it over a period of years, filling notebooks where I'm imagining the story in great detail, and I'm doing that for multiple stories at any given time. When I set out to do a new book, very often I'm looking at the different notebooks in my office and saying, *Which of these am I going to do?*

Once again, you want to take the long view. For sure there are times when a quick Google search will suffice. For example, in the paragraph above, I Googled teaching departments at the Naval War College to write with specificity. Ten seconds. The book that contains the sentence (i.e., the one you are right now holding) relies on twenty-five years of teaching and research. Sometimes we must go deep and remain deep for a long time.

Lastly, I am careful in my own writing practice to keep my research separate from my writing time. When I sit down to draft and commit to two hours, say, of uninterrupted writing time, I will not allow myself to search online for any reason or to double-check any fact. I make a note to return later, but I keep my head down and lay down one word after the next. The internet is a wormhole where time ceases to exist. Once you enter, you may not escape for hours. There is always more to read, more to research, more conversations to be had, places to visit, experiences to be lived. At a certain point, you must stop and commit to the page. Otherwise, research becomes the laundry—just another excuse you make so that you don't have to sit there and write.

36

Crafting Voice

Years ago, when Aidan and Kellen were still little, I lost my voice every February as regularly as Valentine's Day. When I opened my mouth, nothing would come out, no words, no whisper. It often occurred when I was sick, so I didn't worry my inability to speak would be permanent. Instead, I stuffed a notebook in my coat pocket and set off to meet the morning. For the next four days I would play charades with the world, gesturing for my coffee, pointing to the peas I wanted Kellen to eat, writing long notes on the white board in hopes my students would understand the glory of the novel before us. Each day I would grow more depressed, shrink into myself. What had first been a novelty, even a vacation of sorts from parenting and teaching, would start to stifle. Without a voice, I was cut off from everything. Conversations happened all around me while I frantically scrawled notes to make points no longer relevant. I couldn't even call the dentist to complain about the bill.

One February afternoon, Kellen, who at the time was four and not yet a reader, burst into tears when they were unable to decipher my gesture for "get dressed."

"Just use your regular voice, Mama," Kellen cried. "Talk regular."

I couldn't even explain why that was impossible.

Voice is one of the most vital yet ephemeral qualities of writing. We can't point to it on the page, pin it down, say that here, right here, in the way this sentence runs or in this choice of words or in this use of detail, we have voice. Rather, we note its absence by the distance we feel from the writer, from the subject, or from the words on the page; we feel cut off.

In some ways, voice is best defined by what it is not. Voice is not point of view, although the two are related. When we ask about a writer's voice, we aren't asking about the vantage from which a story is narrated—first or second or third person. We might be asking about the intimacy of that point of view, a distinction Dinty Moore makes, but voice and point of view aren't interchangeable. Voice is also not tone or the emotional stance of the narrator toward the material: angry, ironic, remote. A chosen tone may help register the voice, but, again, it isn't the same thing as voice. Nor is it style. An essay can have beautiful, lyrical language and syntax and be devoid of voice. Voice isn't about narrative perspective either—Virginia Woolf's "I now/I then" distinction. Because the narrator tells the story from different perspectives—as a child, then as an adult—doesn't mean the voice changes. The voice remains the same; the perspective switches. Finally, the voice of a piece does not align neatly with the voice of the narrator or a character in a story. Voice doesn't inhabit a pronoun. The speaking "I" in a memoir or essay doesn't provide the voice, or at least not entirely. When we talk about voice, we mean the voice of the writer, the one crafting the narrator, the sentences, the deeper subject. And you can't point to a paragraph or a detail or a line of dialogue and say, there, that is the writer's voice. It exists behind the writing, infusing the language.

Thankfully, while voice may be impossible to point to on the page, it is not impossible to practice. Like all other aspects of writing, voice is a made thing. You don't "find" your voice; you make it. While the intimacy of a chosen point of view or an author's style or tone is important to voice, the real work of creating strong voice is work that takes place off the page. It requires focusing on two aspects of writing: internalization of subject and vulnerability in approach.

When we say a piece has a strong voice, what we are really saying is that the writer fully understands their subject. Not cerebrally but internally, even bodily. It is not enough to research your past—if you are writing memoir—or your subject—if you are writing a short story about rock hounds. Well-researched pieces are often devoid of voice. Think of a text book. To fully understand a subject means to let that subject inhabit you, to live with it, sleep with it, fully know it not in terms of fact but in terms of complication. Only when you fully understand a subject—why your parents' divorce hurt so much when you were twelve or the chemical process of radioactive decay—does that confidence translate to voice on the page.

Whenever I teach voice, I rely on Brian Doyle's essay "Leap." When initially approached about writing a piece in response to 9/11, Doyle is said to have replied to the magazine editor, "No, there is nothing to write. The only thing to say is nothing. Bow your head in prayer and pray whatever prayers you pray. There is nothing to say." He felt the subject was not his own, was not his to write about. At least not initially. But the events of 9/11 would not leave him, and he began to realize that as a writer the only way he could assemble a life post 9/11 was through meeting the event on the page.

In less than 600 words, he tackles one of the greatest tragedies in US history. Three thousand people died. Our way of reckoning time and place forever altered by one morning. What can Doyle say in response? He does not live in New York, was, like most of us, hundreds of miles away. Isn't nothing the only response? How would he have begun?

With falling bodies, I imagine, with the newspaper accounts of blood-filled air. I imagine those bodies kept him awake, that they stalked his sleep. I imagine he couldn't put the bodies down, that he hauled them to the shower in the morning, to work, and home again, that the bodies piled behind his students when he conferenced with him, that he tucked the bodies into bed at night with his children. Until one morning he realized he wasn't sure where his body ended and theirs began. They became his body. They inhabited one another. I imagine it was at that point he began the piece. But not with writing or at least not only with writing. He finds his way into the story not by retelling an event we saw repeated again and again on our televisions but by going to the library, to the archives, learning what he could of the people who leaped to their deaths. He researches the science of falling bodies, the names of the dead. He reads first-person accounts, perhaps interviews witnesses, maybe stands in the middle of New York and looks up into an empty sky. He puts his body in motion (archival and living research) to understand theirs. And the result of that work—physical work, legwork, as well as reflective work—is an essay that draws us in at the first word and never lets us go. His voice is quiet and confident, as well as urgent and pained, but most importantly it's there. The writer is there, even though the first person initially is not. The writer is behind the prose, leading us through his understanding of the disaster. It is because he has so deeply explored his subject—literally in primary- and secondary-source material, as well as reflectively in the way he has carried the piece with him through the days—that we recognize an author, one with authority over what he writes. We hear him speaking to us, know he embodies each of the 600 words.

Doyle's actual body, his "I," does not appear until late in the piece, but it is at that moment that he names his stake in this story, brings forth the sleep-shattered "I." In revealing his investment in the subject, his humanity, we see the second element necessary for crafting voice: the writer's vulnerability. At the moment the "I" enters, the prose changes, signifying the shift in responsibility for the story. He moves from a newspaper accounting of the event—simple sentences pierced by facts, quote-filled lines reporting what witnesses saw—and moves into the lyric, a space defined by emotion rather than reason, a space defined by association rather than chronology, where his sentences tumble across one another, falling like so many bodies down the page, only to topple into a heap at the end, leaving his body holding onto their bodies "against horror and loss and death."

The form of his piece, the way he strings his sentences together, his diction, his images all conspire to name his stake in the story: the human capacity for love. And we join with him in his whispered prayer, unable to ever see the events of that day in the same way again. We now hold those bodies in our own because Doyle was first unable to lay them aside. And because we know that a real body, a person whose humanity replicates our own, is writing, is behind these words on the page, we listen. We hear the writer's voice—not some projection, some flimsy prop—but a person who has been changed by his subject, embodies his subject, just the way his voice embodies the prose.

Every piece of writing relies on voice. It's what lends the work urgency, what keeps the reader's attention. When the voice of an essay is vibrant and strong, the words cannot remain unheard.

37

It's Not about Cake

In this chapter, I want to bring a few ideas together by offering a way to think about writing, and art more generally, in visual terms. Basically, any piece of art, is working simultaneously in two directions. Some part of a work is in pursuit of the horizontal: what is happening in the manifest, material world (i.e., scene, physical detail, dialogue, etc.). And some part of a work is invested in the vertical: considering what it means to be human, or what the purpose of life is, or why we are here. Sometimes a piece of art will emphasize the horizontal line (think *Hunger Games* or a Constable landscape) and sometimes the vertical line prevails (think Basquiat or Woolf's essay "Death of a Moth"), but I would argue that all art falls somewhere along this axis. And all art must ascend, to some extent, the vertical line, because that is where the reader will connect with what is happening in the story or poem. We have seen this in terms of the musing voice as well as significant detail—craft elements that open portals to the vertical line (what I have been terming deeper subject up to this point).

As we saw earlier in the book, the metaphors we use in everyday language reveal much about who we are as both individuals and communities, as well as what we value. Sometimes we are aware of their magical powers. For example, when we say we need to "iron out the details," we know we mean that we will produce a plan that is as unwrinkled as a white Oxford pressed by steam (a metaphor becomes a dead metaphor when the use of the metaphor no longer conjures an image—when we don't actually envision an iron when we say we will iron out the details. So this may be a dead metaphor, but we understand its original meaning). Sometimes, we are unaware of what a metaphor carries. For example, when we say something is "beyond the pale," we rarely think of the pale as a geographic place that stands outside legal jurisdiction, one demarcated, initially, by pales or stakes to physically guard the civilized from the unacceptable, the barbaric, or indecent. Metaphors are one of the primary ways a writer leaves the horizontal of storytelling and enters the vertical realm of the less easily said. Metaphors multiply possibility. They untether language from the concrete (the horizontal) and allow a four-letter word like, say, cake to hold loss, suffering, disappointment, and pain in its crumb.

Briefly, "Cake" is an essay by Debra Gwartney about a single piece of chocolate cake that sits wrapped in plastic on the edge of the kitchen counter. Trapped and precarious. Neither the counter nor the kitchen nor the piece of German chocolate cake belongs to a young Gwartney. Instead, she imagines that this single piece of cake in her friends' kitchen is being saved for their sweet child who sleeps amid "planets and stars in dreamy shades of blue" in a themed bedroom down the hall. Her husband remains in the living room, laughing with their friends, while Gwartney stands in the kitchen knowing that she is pregnant with her fourth baby at a moment in her life when she was just about to pack her three other children and leave her husband. At twenty-eight, her life has passed her by. She is as stained as the dress that she wears, the one spotted with gravy. Like the cake, she is trapped, trapped by the desire that began her troubles when she became pregnant as a teen, and trapped, too, by three children who need her. Reclaiming want for a moment, Gwartney grabs the piece of cake, "like a swimmer gasping for air," and stuffs the wedge into her pregnant body without even stopping to chew.

Just recently, I was guest teaching in Aidan's AP Literature class and we were studying "Cake." I went around the room of thirty students and asked each of them to provide one word for what the cake represented. I received thirty different answers—ranging from loneliness and desire to the author herself. Every response was right, and, because of her elegant understanding of metaphor, Gwartney can claim every one of those readings. The cake is not just cake. It becomes the portal to the vertical, a place where sorrow and loss and grief dwell, joy and pleasure, too, all those experiences that are held in common by human beings but are incapable of being fully expressed.

All art strikes a balance between the time it dwells in the horizontal and the time it spends in the vertical. In writing, when we talk about the vertical we primarily use geographical language to explain how a writer moves there—we might talk about taking a piece deeper or we might talk about taking a piece to a higher level—but either way we are describing the need for all writing to move beyond the literal, the concrete, the chronological. We are also, in our choice of directional language, pointing to our understanding that meaning resides outside/above/below the words on the page. Hemingway's famous six-word story—"For sale: baby shoes. Never worn"—punches us in the gut because we are reading underneath the words. We bring our own experience of sadness into the empty spaces between "shoes" and "never" and "worn." The actual words don't wring our heart. What we intuit between the words is what does. It is not happenstance that we think of the deeper work of art as a vertical dimension that operates above and below the concrete. Below is the space of the subconscious, murky, dark, and full of possibility. Above is the space of what in yoga is termed the *sattvic*, the pure, essential, the sacred. Neither space is fully available to us in our existence as embodied beings, but both spaces inform the choices that we make.

The vertical is what allows the reader to connect to the piece. I did not become pregnant as a teen. I have never stolen a piece of cake from a friend's kitchen counter. But I do know loss and sorrow and how one can feel alone even when surrounded by others. Gwartney isn't writing about cake. If she were, she would have written a cookbook. Instead, she is trying to convey an alienation and sorrow that is much too expansive, gripping, and complex to name in language—no matter how many words she uses. The story of standing in the kitchen is just that: the *story*. It is horizontal. I came to the party, went to the kitchen, saw a piece of cake, and ate it. The *deeper subject* is loss itself. As a reader, you can become entranced by a story (think of your friend running up to you and saying, "You're never going to guess what just happened on the bus!" That's a story you want to hear. And you are expecting some good drama). But, as a reader, you will not *carry* a story unless it has a deeper subject, unless it points to something larger than simply the time a person ate a piece of cake. Story and deeper subject. Or, another way you will hear this relationship between the horizontal and vertical described is the "what" and the "so what." The "what" is the narrative or subject or story and the "so what" is what the writer wants to say above or below (take your pick) the story itself.

Your writing must contain a deeper subject, even if you are pursuing a largely horizontal line. Novels like *Harry Potter* or *The Shining* still contain deeper subjects even as they entertain or frighten. If they didn't, they wouldn't remain. That's the magic of the vertical. It is a doorway that you, as a writer, enter, but then it becomes *the* doorway through which your readers will pass. Think of the books you carry with you, that private library full of characters and lines and scenes that return to you time and again. You carry those books or poems because the doorway the writer has created is one you recognize and understand. The work resonates with you. You recognize yourself or some aspect of the human condition underneath or between or behind the actual words.

Your job, as a writer, or at least one of your jobs, is to determine what your deeper subject is. In other words, you have to figure out what your story or essay or poem is actually about. It's never about cake. Writers discover their deeper subject. They have to mine their own work to find it because the deeper subject is so deep, so far beneath/above/below/between their words that even they don't know it at the start. They write their way toward it, each sentence like a flashlight directing them further down. Put another way, you cannot know your deeper subject before you begin. If you do, you are in trouble. Your work will arrive didactic and heavy handed. The reader will feel like they are being beaten by the theme or idea. Often, new writers want to write smart, political stories that take on the great themes of inequality or injustice. They write an overtly environmental story or a story that dismantles patriarchy from the beginning. The reader wants to find the deeper subject on their own (remember, thirty different responses to what the piece of cake represents), and the *only* way the reader will be allowed to discover a deeper subject is if they, like the writer, are encouraged to explore.

You actually want to begin with a mess, unsure of what you are writing. You begin at the bottom so you, too, can try to make sense of your characters' predicament or your speaker's lament. You do not want to know what your story or essay or memory is about. You write to discover, and then you replicate that journey for your reader.

That raises the question of how you figure out your deeper subject. Because while you can't know when you begin, you have to know by the time you end. Here is where meta writing comes in. Meta writing is simply writing about writing. You writing about your own writing. Toward the middle of your project, your writing notebook will naturally move from taking notes and brainstorming and writing prompts into a space where you can think through on the page what it is you are doing in your work. There are two questions you can ask yourself at the start of each day of journaling. In one sentence can you name the "what" of your poem, essay, or story? For example, I am writing about the time I stole a piece of candy from the Brach's pick-a-mix display. Or I am writing about a character whose father died suddenly of a stomach infection while they were getting a massage. That's the easy part. Now you spend the rest of your writing time trying to do that same kind of concise writing with your deeper subject. Ask yourself, on the top of the page, what I am really writing about is ____. At first, it will take you pages and pages to figure out what you are actually exploring. Each day as you tackle the question, you will write yourself closer to the answer. Eventually, and this could be weeks, months, years down the road, you will be able to articulate in a single sentence what you are really writing about. When you are able to do that, you know you are close to being "done," whatever that might mean. For example, I am really writing about the way the body betrays us. Or, I am writing about a grief that never ends.

One more point. We write toward our deeper subject as we draft. If you are unsure of what your poem or story or essay might actually be about, pay attention to where you end up. Most often, the final line is actually the place we need to begin the work. We figure out, fifteen pages into a story, what the stakes are for our characters or for ourselves. That's because writing is fundamentally a way of knowing. The important thing to keep in mind is that once we know what we are writing about, we then have to return to the beginning and revise with the deeper subject in mind. More on that in the chapter on chopping limbs. Understand, here, that a good place to know where you need to begin is by seeing where you end.

38

Drop the Knife

Like many mindfulness paths, yoga offers an ethical code to guide those who practice as they move off the mat and into their lives. They are called the *yamas* and *niyamas*. I think of them as the five things not to do (hurt, lie, steal, overindulge, and covet) and the five things to seek (purity, contentment, self-discipline, self-study, and surrender). In systems of Indian philosophy, the item that comes first in a list is considered the most important (as well as the item that comes last in the list), so the order always tells us something. In the *yamas* and the *niyamas*, the practice of *ahimsā*, or nonviolence, arrives first. Most would say that if you follow *ahimsā*, the other *yamas* and *niyamas* become unnecessary. Everything you need to know about living ethically can be found in this one practice.

Whenever I share the fact that nonviolence is the most important of the *yamas* and *niyamas* with my yoga students, I can feel them release a collective sigh. I imagine they were worried I would tell them that the most important ethical practice was finding enlightenment or giving up caffeine. *Ahimsā* appears easy by comparison; after all, none of us are really violent. We don't make a practice of punching people or running them down with our cars or biting children. We are all basically kind. When was the last time you actually struck another being physically? Decades ago, I would imagine, if ever. So when we learn that *ahimsā* is the single most important ethical practice we can follow in our lives, we often feel like we have that one covered. No problem. And our angel wings sprout from our scapula.

Of course, it's not that simple. We have to move beyond physical acts of violence and consider the much more subtle actions we take against others and, here is the rub, ourselves. As Deborah Adele reminds us, "our ability to be nonviolent is directly related to our ability to be nonviolent within ourselves." Too often when we hear about violence, we think about external actions being done by an oppressor against a victim. And those acts do take place. But what we need to consider is the tiny beatings enacted upon ourselves all day long. The ways in which we tell ourselves that we aren't good enough or smart enough, that we are unworthy, we are abandoned, we are selfish, we are pathetic, or we are losers. This kind of self-talk—these daily bruisings, cuttings, and beatings—can be hard to detect. Sure, we have a moment where we look in the mirror and don't like what we see. But what about when you wake up and see the pile of laundry at the foot of your bed and abrade yourself for not doing it the night before. Or what about the silent condemnation you make against yourself when you don't get up in time to exercise. Or the shaming you use as a strap against your flesh when you eat a second helping at dinner or a bowl of ice cream. Or the way in which you carry around your loneliness and tell yourself that you aren't lovable. If you are like me, these acts of violence happen all day long and without stop. They are subtle, quiet, almost undetectable, and we rarely label them as violence. But how we talk to ourselves on the inside is how we meet the world. There is no difference. Adele writes, "The color of paint inside the can is the color that whatever we paint becomes." You cannot expect a can of red paint to cover the walls of the world in blue. Our violence against ourselves seeps out. It cannot be contained. And then we mark those around us, not with our fists but with our words.

The great poet Hafiz writes a poem about a woman who wants to know how to find God. You can substitute Love or Beauty or Oneness here. The question is basically how do we become our best and highest selves. The poet responds, "My dear, they have dropped the knife. Someone / who knows God has dropped the cruel knife // that most so often use upon their tender self / and others." Drop the knife. So simple and yet so hard. The cuts we have made, intimate and deep. It's why affirmations so often don't work. I am sure you have heard at some point in your life that you can counter the mental monster in your head by practicing affirmations: I am good. I am loved. I am whole. But for me, my mental monsters are so tyrannical that they shred those tiny (though true) affirmations to bits. I hear the monsters mocking my attempts to reclaim worth.

Instead, I am going to suggest the practice of *metta*, or loving-kindness, and combine *metta* with breath work. The violence we enact against ourselves will not go away overnight. I have made it my life's work to quiet my inner demons rather than thinking I can banish them entirely. I would encourage you to practice *metta* with the same goal in mind—a gentling rather than an eradication. We want to feel successful—otherwise we will just create another whip to self-flagellate.

Come to a comfortable pose and begin your three-part breath. Once you have established the fullness of your lungs, then move to a four- and six-count breath, slowing everything down. There are many versions of *metta*, and I am just offering the version that I was taught long ago. To begin, bring before your mind's eye a stranger that you have passed today. Maybe someone you noticed driving in a car, or someone you saw walking down the street, or out of a building. Or maybe the cashier at the grocery store, the neighbor down the street, the cane-aided human who walks their three elderly beagles every morning no matter the temperature. Pick someone you don't know but someone whom you can see easily. Hold them before you.

Inhale slowly. On your exhalation, say to them, "May you be free of suffering."

Inhale again and exhale, saying, "May you have peace."

Inhale again and exhale, saying, "May you find joy."

Do this again, wishing the same three things for the individual. Try to really visualize the person, maybe even imagine a string or a beam of light running from your heart to theirs. Wish for this total stranger some relief from the burdens that they carry. Give them the greatest gifts we have to give as human beings—your time and your attention. Hold them.

Next, bring before you someone you love. Someone maybe you know is suffering. Maybe someone you haven't seen for a while or someone you just saw at breakfast. At this time, don't bring before you someone with whom your relationship is vexed. Bring a simple love, a clear love, an easy love to your mind's eye. Wish for them the same three things, letting the exhalation carry your love, your *metta*, to them no matter where they are or if they are living or dead.

May you be free of suffering.

May you have peace.

May you find joy.

Sit with them for a few breaths and then let them go.

Now bring before you someone who is difficult. You don't need to pick your archenemy or the person who has wronged you the most. It is so hard to feel love for those who have hurt us. Baby steps here. Just bring someone before you who is less easy to love. Someone who tests your patience or your limits. Someone whose own suffering turns them into a creature harder to meet. Wish for them the same three things. Wish it for them without condition. Wish it for them purely because all human beings, all beings on the planet, fundamentally deserve to be loved. Wish far past any wrongs they have done you. Wish it for the part of them that is, and will always be, pure and good and whole, even if that part is buried deep.

The final move is the most difficult. If you found it challenging to extend your heart toward someone who is less than perfect, now you have to face the biggest monster, the meanest bully, the one who has, possibly, caused the most pain to you in your life, and that is you. At this moment, bring before you an image of yourself at the age of five. Maybe take your kindergarten picture as your guide or any other photo of yourself at a young age. Hold that child before you. See their eyes. Notice their smile and baby teeth. See their tiny nose and soft chin. Look at their little outfit, the tiny T-shirt. Wish for them the same things.

May you be free of suffering.

May you have peace.

May you find joy.

Do it again and again and again and again. Look into your child self's eyes. See how small you were. How little your hands. How short your legs. Notice how open your face is, unguarded, and innocent. See your fragility. See your beauty and trust in the world. See how your skin has not been scarred, your trust has not been broken, your belief that the world will hold and protect you is still intact. If, at the age of five, this was not true for you, then, first, I just want to say I am sorry. Too many break too early. And I wish that the world were more kind. If by five, your childhood was already taken, then go further back. A baby picture. Before language. Just out of the womb.

May you be free of suffering.

May you have peace.

May you find joy.

Say these things to your child self again and again. That child is still within you. They have never left. How could they? They are you. Where would they have gone? They are still there. You can send them love. You can assure your child self that they are going to be okay. And, in assuring them, in taking care of them, in sending them love, you are also tending your adult self. You are changing the story inside your head, just slightly, just for a moment, but feel the light pour in through the crack you have just made. Let it expand your heart.

39

The Body, The House

The brain develops in the womb as it did during evolution. The first part of the brain to form is the most primitive part, the most deep-rooted, the most ancient. Some call this our reptilian brain. The second part to form is the limbic system (including both the amygdala and the thalamus), which categorizes input and maintains the relation between the self and its immediate environment. Together, trauma expert Bessel van der Kolk writes, the reptilian and the mammalian brains create our "emotional brain." The emotional brain stands in contrast to, though not in opposition of, the frontal lobes, where all our thinking takes place. The rational brain is what makes us humans, allows us to use language and generate abstract thought. It is where most of us would say our identity exists, the thinking part. Every experience that we have in our lives, though, must pass through the pre-verbal part of our brain first before it moves to the rational. If the limbic system—van der Kolk calls the limbic system the smoke detector—decides that a situation is dangerous (and remember the limbic is making this decision without the aid of thinking—it "sees" a coiled line, codes snake, and our bodies jump long before the rational considers size, length, probability), it tells the body to fight, to freeze, or to flee. Trauma is the result of an experience being labeled by the limbic as threatening so it is never allowed to make its way to the rational brain, where it can be sorted and held by language. Instead the trauma haunts, remaining outside any story we can tell of the experience. What it haunts is the body.

Van der Kolk titles his book on trauma *The Body Keeps the Score* to highlight his point that the body, and the body alone, knows what has assailed it, not the head. Trauma is in the tissue, the organs, the nerves. Any attempt at healing, therefore, cannot involve the rational brain because the trauma never made it to that kind of mental awareness. "Trauma," he writes, "is not stored as a narrative with an orderly beginning, middle, and end." Instead, he says, those who have suffered trauma must return to their bodies, must come home to the body they have abandoned or neglected or abused and feel into their bodies and be with their pain. We cannot think our way to healing; we must, in a sense, reincarnate into our healing. And this begins, he says, when we "first agree to exile nothing."

A standard practice in the recovery from trauma is talk therapy, where the one who has survived is given a space where they can finally put words to their experience, revise their past, and claim agency or power over something that has previously only diminished and paralyzed them. Writing as healing works in the same way, except that the writer is both the therapist and the one coming to therapy. Someone who has undergone trauma can write their way to healing by externalizing a story that has, until then, only haunted their bodies. And research demonstrates that writing about horrific events can improve physical and mental health.

But we are also learning how mindfulness practices can create healing without the need to ever have to actually name the trauma. Since Freud, the focus in trauma therapy has been on narrating that which haunts the body. If you can name it, the belief was, then you can move past it. Recently, researchers are discovering that the trauma itself never has to be actually organized into a story. What has to be affirmed is the body's response. How the body feels. In mindfulness—all the breath work we have been doing throughout the book—we are taught to inhabit our bodies and be with whatever our bodies feel. We don't have to solve anything, or change anything, or do anything. We simply descend from our brains into our hearts and sit with whatever arises. "In order to find our voice," Van der Kolk says, "we have to be *in* our bodies—able to access our inner sensations."

We might initially feel that this conversation doesn't apply to us because nothing "traumatic" has happened. My first response is the one the writer Madeleine L'Engle gave to me when I asked her at the age of twenty-two, not yet divorced, and living the dream on the island of Oahu, whether I could be a writer if I hadn't suffered. She replied, "Just keep writing. The suffering will come." Amen, sister. So, if you initially think you don't need to consider the relationship between trauma and art because you live a luck-filled life, I would suggest that you just keep living. Trauma arrives. To be human, the Buddha tells us, is to suffer.

I also think it's important that we understand the ways in which trauma is being redefined these days. Twenty years ago, trauma was equated with acute psychological trauma, enormous events like rape and war that entirely undo a human being. And while, for sure, those kinds of experiences are traumatic, we understand now that trauma—the ways in which the body keeps the score—exceeds the boundaries of these kinds of events. The field of epigenetics, for example, reveals how trauma is handed down almost like eye color on a molecular level. Your body holds the traumas of your ancestors, their anger, their shame, their expulsion, their extinction, their inability to live freely. In addition, your zip code perhaps as much as your genetic code speaks to the trauma your body carries: race, class, gender, and sexuality mark the physical body in often unseen ways. Resmaa Menakem writes,

"What we call out as individual personality flaws, dysfunctional family, or twisted cultural norms are sometimes manifestations of historical trauma." He continues, "If we were born and raised in America," he says. "white-body supremacy and our adaptations to it are in our blood. Our very bodies house the unhealed dissonance and trauma of our ancestors." Like van der Kolk, Menakem asserts that no amount of talk about racism will ever overcome racism because racism resides in our bodies, not our heads. It's cellular. We have to move back into our bodies and feel our discomfort, our fragility, our fears. Finally, much work focuses on micro-aggressions to reveal the ways in which systems of power (white, male, and straight) maintain their advantage not in dramatic ways but in the daily ways that continue their privilege while denying others their dignity and agency. All of these areas of research point us away from acute psychological trauma and toward the trauma of living an ordinary life. They also point us to our bodies.

No one is outside. We all inhabit traumatized bodies. The only difference between the experience of our traumatized bodies is the difference that exists between those who are willing to return to the site of the crime and heal and those who live from the neck up and pretend that everything is just fine. As writers, we cannot choose the second option. For the sake of our characters, for the sake of our deeper subject, for the sake of our art and our own humanity, we must do the work of sitting with our bodies and the sensations that arise. Being able to sit with discomfort and sorrow and pain is difficult, but Menakem tells us that pain is "clean pain." Clean pain is marked by acceptance, while dirty pain is marked by avoidance, denial, and blame. Both hurt, but the first allows for healing.

If this conversation about trauma reminds you of the discussion about creating characters, then you are seeing the connections I have been trying to draw between our role as writers and the way writing allows us to become better human beings. Van der Kolk insists that we exile nothing. In our lives and on the page, we allow contradiction, shame, and sorrow to exist—whether that is in our own bodies or the bodies of our characters. "Hurt people," he tells us, "hurt people." When we alleviate our own pain—by writing and breathing and swaying and feeling—then we will hurt others less often. And that is the best that we can do.

40

Finding Form

When I introduce nonlinearity to my students, I quote Annie Dillard, who says, "original writing fashions a form." She adds, "It grows cell to cell, hole to bough to twig to leaf." The form itself carries meaning in its structure. I want my students to understand that, like all the arts from dance to pottery, form and content are wed in writing. Or at least they should be. The form a writer utilizes—from linear to nonlinear and everything in between—should depend on what the writer is trying to say, the subject of the piece. The trick, I tell my students, is not one of choosing a form the way one might choose an ice cream topping. Form is not a condiment added for flavor. Rather, the trick is one of perception, recognizing the form as it emerges from the ideas. And such perception, such nimbleness of mind, comes with time and experience. The more exposure a writer has to the different constellations ideas can assume, the more readily they see the form their subject requires.

As I described earlier, we tend to think both life and narrative unfold along a chronological path—first this happened, then this, and then this—and we often assume that our poem, essay, or story should proceed linearly. But linearity should not and cannot be the default form for our writing. Just like setting or diction or character, *form is a choice*, one that writers must make. To make that choice necessitates an understanding of the limits and possibilities found in both linear and nonlinear writing.

In *Narrative Design*, Madison Smartt Bell offers a useful way to think about narrative structure, providing a continuum of sorts, with all prose falling somewhere along the continuum and no piece occupying either end entirely. On one end of the continuum is what Bell calls "linear design," narratives that "start at the beginning, traverse some sort of middle, and stop at the end." Linear narratives, Bell tells us, are chronologically bound. Events progress over time in a cause-and-effect fashion. They are timebound and sequential—if not entirely then at least in terms of how they gain their narrative momentum. Something happens because something else has happened—a domino effect. Linear stories build, climax, and then end. In Western literature, linear stories are the ones that have been historically honored and valued. Aristotle writes in *Poetics* that beauty in drama results from the "proper arrangement of the incidents," an arrangement that creates a whole, "what has a beginning and middle and end."

Linear design, though, assures more than just the inherent logic of the subject under study. Linearity suggests that the subject or the experience has been integrated, understood, and can be rendered as complete. The writer is implying in their choice of form that the parts add up to a whole and that the whole is best understood in relation to time. Because we understand chronology on an almost cellular level—when we wake in the morning we orient ourselves to time immediately by determining the day of the week—when we meet a linear story it feels "natural." While we may have other work to do in order to derive meaning, the task of determining how disparate parts are related to the greater whole has been done for us by the writer. Time is the controlling force; chronology is the line we should follow.

But linear narratives are limited, as all writers quickly come to understand. They are predictable in terms of structure; they require large amounts of space to tell; and, because they are organized in relation to time, they fail to reflect actual lived experience. While we might tell the story of what happened on the way to work that day as a story with a beginning, middle, and end, our actual experience of going to work was not nearly so logical. To start, we are rarely only doing one thing. And even if we are, our minds are rarely focused entirely on that one thing. We are walking intersections of past experiences, current impressions, and future projections. Nothing in our day comes close to being linear. So the linear, as a narrative structure, in many ways is a lie.

Bell offers as the other end of the continuum "modular design." For Bell, "modular design allows the writer to throw off the burden of chronology as much as possible." The writer no longer binds themselves to chronology or a cause-and-effect understanding of their subject. They work by association instead, moving from, say, image to image, rather than moment to moment. Nonlinear form occupies the far end of the narrative structure spectrum, the moment before prose falls over into poetry, no longer bound by sentence but instead by line.

Often rendered in chunks of text on the page with white space in between, nonlinear forms behave like poetry, leaping from one image-laden paragraph to the next, asking readers to do the work of navigating the white space. Nonlinear forms, like mosaics, are only whole at a great distance, a point Bell makes when describing modular design. More importantly, any sense of understanding or wholeness is temporary at best. The subject, the writer implies with the nonlinear form, cannot be held; it slips and falls between our fingers, tiny bits of prose raining down like sand.

Because nonlinear form resides outside of time, privileging relationships instead, it is much harder to read, as well as to write. The further from the troll-like narrative line a writer moves, the more work they have to do to bind the piece together. If a writer abandons the driving force of chronology, they better have something equally compelling to offer in its place. Typically, again, these are images or metaphors, the common currency of poetry. Still, a reader must struggle when reading a nonlinear essay or story. Brenda Miller writes in "A Braided Heart" that the form "has a tendency toward fragmentation that invites the reader into [the] gaps." In those empty spaces, represented literally by the white space on the page, meaning resides, or at least a hint at meaning, a nod toward understanding. What is so compelling about nonlinear work is that the meaning derived by the reader is often one filled with questions, hesitation, and unknowing. Unlike linear structure, which suggests to the reader that the subject has a beginning, middle, and end, a nonlinear structure implies the subject cannot be fully known at all. We can move in a particular, though often circular, direction, through the accretion of image, but we rarely live happily ever after.

Broadly speaking, a writer will either be sustaining the narrative line or deserting it in favor of association. And that choice should arise organically from the writer's relationship to their material. In fact, the basic decision between linear or nonlinear will tell us how the writer views the subject before we meet the first word.

Sometimes a writer wants their page to resemble more clearly their own journey into a subject or a character's experience of their day. They might choose a nonlinear form. Take, for example, Deborah Tall's *A Family of Strangers*, a nonlinear memoir about her family that traces the legacy of genocide. She is asking what happens to Jews long after Hitler's demise, and the answer is, not surprisingly, complicated. Her memoir arrives in short bursts of prose that circle in ever-maddening rings. We don't understand, because she doesn't understand, because the slaughter and black holes created by such destruction are ultimately unknowable. The aftermath of the Holocaust is not meant to be understood, to be held, to have a beginning, middle, and an end. Its effects never end; they go on and on. The nonlinear form is the only possible choice for Tall. To write linearly would be to ignore her history and experience.

Survivors of trauma might choose a nonlinear form, sensing once again that knowledge of such an event is impossible. Toni Morrison's novel *Beloved* changes point of view and narrative style without warning, juxtaposes the past and the present, and relies on ambiguity to underscore the generational legacy of trauma and its often invisible and insidious harm. While a novel like Michael Cunningham's *The Hours* works to reveal how social conventions destroy lives across time and space by weaving in and out of three separate but connected narratives. The relationship between trauma and the nonlinear form is particularly tight because, as we just read, traumatic memory is held imagistically in our brains rather than narratively. Biology creates a natural affinity between traumatic memory and the associational nature of nonlinear form.

Those on the outside of dominant society—those marginalized by race or class or gender or sexuality—might choose a nonlinear form because their experiences cannot be narrated within the confines of a narrative structure promulgated by those in power. Or a writer might use a nonlinear form, pulling a personal strand through their research, because they understand that all knowledge is subjective and they want to highlight the porosity between knower and known. A writer might choose a nonlinear form for any number of reasons; the point to remember, though, is that it is an act of deciding. Or perhaps, more accurately, an act of discerning. A writer must see their subject, inhabit their subject, well enough to see the form that will carry their meaning. In the end, it might be linear, but that would be because a linear form is the right form and not because it is the default form. Every form brings gains and losses. There is no "best" form. And it may take a writer many attempts before understanding the surest form for their deeper subject. Once found, though, it should appear to the reader that no other form was possible, that this story had to be rendered this way and no other. Only then are form and content truly working at their highest level.

PART THREE

Distillation—*Recaka*

41

Winnowing

In this third part of the book, we turn to the exhalation as well as the act of revision. If the inhalation teaches us gratitude and points to the fullness of our lives, then the exhalation tells us how to let everything go. I remember a time when I was seeing a wonderful acupuncturist named Billie Arlt, who practiced her craft in the tiny town of Preston, Idaho, amid rangeland, and mountains, and churchgoing folk. She had just finished placing needles in my cheeks and around my eyes and was about to let me "simmer" in all the energy being released when she said, "None of us are making it out of here alive." While I have heard versions of the expression since then, that was the first time I really saw that deep down inside I had some crazy hope that by doing everything right, never making a mistake, always succeeding that I would somehow cheat death—not on any rational level but way deep down. What other reason could I give for living life as if it were a race and wanting very much to win first place.

Nothing remains. Nothing. Not even the mountains that rise up around me where I live, or the hard edges of the continents, or the love I have for my children. Our culture tries to convince us otherwise—promises that we can live longer, live better, that forty is the new twenty. Our economic systems suggest that we can own—among other things—the planet itself. This is my house, my yard, my car, my baby, my idea, my body. But it will all pass away. All of it. So every time we assert our youth, every time we assert our ownership, every time we say this is mine and not yours, we are fighting against what is fundamentally true. And that creates more suffering. The Buddha lays it out very clearly in his Four Noble Truths: the only way for our suffering to end is to surrender and let go. To be at peace with loss. And the exhalation of our breath teaches us how to take a step in that direction some 22,000 times a day.

I invite you to sit with your exhalation the next time you breathe with intention. Return to your four- and six-count breath, but keep your focus on following the exhalation down your body. While the inhalation moves up and out (fullness, creation), the exhalation takes us down and in. When you view the breath as a funnel, you can feel the inhalation expanding at the collarbones and widening at the very top of the inhalation, but when you follow the exhalation back down, the energy narrows and you eventually arrive at the very bottom of the exhalation, deep in the belly. A pinpoint. Exhalation is a winnowing, a lessening. And what your body is letting go of every single time is the very substance that you need to live. Just think about that. Breath keeps us alive, yet our bodies release the breath and trust that a new breath will arrive. That is a powerful lesson in letting go. We are shown, time and again, that surrender does not mean destitution and poverty; surrender does not mean that you will forever be without; surrender just opens space for you to receive what arrives next. We are being taught with every out-breath to trust that the world will take care of us, that we will be given what we need. We only have to let go.

If you follow the exhalation long enough, you can start to experience how the exhalation actually carves space in your body. Physically, the exhalation is removing carbon dioxide, so it is literally carrying waste away. But we would be foolish, I think, to attend only to the physical, especially when it comes to the breath which is simultaneously both gross and subtle. I think of the exhalation as excavating the body or mining the body, clearing channels so that the next inhalation travels even further, irrigates even more. The deeper we exhale, the more room we create for the next inhalation. So allow each exhalation to tunnel further in your body; see if you can exhale all the way down to your toes.

After you have deepened your exhalation, try to experience the breath as *beginning* on the exhalation rather than the inhalation. Your breath won't change in terms of form, but your experience of your breath will alter. Begin, then, with a six-count exhalation and end with a four-count inhalation. Let surrender and letting go be what guides your body. Each exhalation clears new space, new pathways, new channels by a deepening commitment to loss. Feel how powerful it is to lead with surrender.

The same is true in our writing. In *The Writing Life*, Annie Dillard gives this advice:

> One of the things I know about writing is this: spend it all, shoot it, play it, lose it, all, right away, every time. Do not hoard what seems good for a later place in the book or for another book; give it, give it all, give it now. The impulse to save something good for a better place later is the signal to spend it now. Something more will arise for later, something better. These things fill from behind, from beneath, like well water. Similarly, the impulse to keep to yourself what you have learned is not only shameful, it is destructive. Anything you do not give freely and abundantly becomes lost to you. You open your safe and find ashes.

This is what it means to allow the exhalation to guide our writing practice. Spend it all now. As artists, we don't want to replicate the world around us, one bent on keeping and having, claiming and owning, protecting and hoarding. Such a stance is outright hostile to the idea of creation—how can we create when we are busy holding on to what we already have? Instead, we follow the lesson found in the breath and learn to let go, trust that another inhalation will arrive.

Dillard is encouraging us, specifically, not to save words and ideas for later, not to write inside a model of scarcity. Trust, she says, that "things fill from behind, from beneath, like well water." There is no best idea, no last idea. We don't hoard metaphors or cache similes. We spend it all each and every time. Surrender in our writing applies to the entire process—letting go of everything, including any results. The more we can release in our practice (release expectation, evaluation, fear, longing), the more space we create for the new to enter. Time spent judging, time spent comparing, time spent saving or protecting or claiming is time not spent on making. There are only so many hours in the day, fewer that you can dedicate solely to your craft. Spend them on the exhalation.

Often at the beginning of a yoga class, when I have students focus on their breath and on the exhalation in particular, I encourage them to allow the exhalation to take whatever it is they don't want to carry into their practice. It can be something small—the argument they had with their partner that morning over whose turn it was to take the garbage out—or it can be large—a miscarriage, a death, divorce, loss of work. We can allow all of that to ride the exhalation out of the body. Some of it we may need to pick back up after class or after we are done writing for the day. We all must carry a certain amount of pain. But we can choose what we want to hold and how we want to hold it, and there is every chance it will be lighter because we set it down for a moment.

The exhalation does not protect us from loss; it teaches us how to work with it. As writers, we want to learn what we can from the out-breath. As humans, our mental health and happiness depend on how well we can let go, adapt, surrender. Take some time to inhabit your exhalation. Learn how it travels in your body. Watch the way it returns you again and again to ground zero, how it burrows its way into the stuck places in your body, heart, and mind. Allow the exhalation to ferry away all that you do not need. And trust the next inhalation, the next sentence, the next project, the next idea to arrive.

42

See the Wolf

When Aidan and Kellen were little, we used to play a game called Telestrations. A cross between the Telephone game and Pictionary, the game involved each player sketching a word or phrase they had been given and then passing their sketch on to the next person who would decide what they thought the drawing resembled and redraw it for the next person. At the end, each player would review the series of sketches out loud, thereby providing all sorts of hilarity as "doggy bag" devolved into "poop purse." We played Telestrations a lot, mostly because Kellen liked it, and there were few board games Kellen enjoyed. Naturally artistic, they were also very good at Telestrations. If I sat next to Kellen, I always knew exactly what they had sketched, even when they were no more than five or six years old. My drawings, on the other hand, single-handedly assured that no phrase would make it through unscathed. No matter how long I spent on my tiny sketch, my dog resembled my elephant, as well as my human, a house, a watering can, and a wagon. Good thing I was born to write and not draw.

Since the game depends on people with poor drawing skills to make a mess of things, just as the Telephone game is no fun if the whispered phrase survives the circle, I was happy to be mocked by my family for a car that had wheels twice the size of its body. But I also began to watch more closely at what Kellen was doing that made their drawings so recognizable. It was, I understood, a way of seeing the subject and understanding its fundamental attributes. For example, when drawing a wolf, Kellen seemed to intuit which characteristics set the wolf apart from mammals in general and dogs more specifically. Maybe it was in the ears, or the line of the jaw, or the way the animal held its head. Whatever it was, Kellen could see the essential quality and then replicate it. That is the kind of vision that becomes necessary when you move from drafting to revising. You must be able to determine the fundamental shape of your piece, know your work with such clarity that you have a firm sense of what needs to remain—those pointed ears, the narrow pupils, the exposed neck—and what needs to go—the rat running between the paws, the mountains in the back, the color you chose for fur.

You have spent the last many chapters writing from both heart and gut. You have, I hope, delayed the entrance of the mind and its ability to categorize, label, separate, and define. Instead, you have put the blinders on, cottoned your ears, muted your devices, and laid down one word after another, every day, every single day, even when you didn't want to, even when it felt hard, hopeless, inane, even when it was snowing, or you ate too many doughnuts, or your mother had a plumbing disaster, or your father needed someone to mow the lawn or find a flashlight or fish with him, still you showed up and, importantly, you invited no one else to the party. You have been relentless. You have not waited for the muse; you have not looked outside yourself for validation or help; you have done the work.

The work itself may be the place where you are happiest.

This may be the writing that you are called to do.

You may decide the act of writing is what matters the most, the joy of telling a story, the satisfaction that comes from alliteration or a well-turned line of poetry. In fact, I hope you do. You will be happier. Any sorrow or sadness in the life of one born to write only comes from the moment the writer decides to share their work. You can release yourself from that suffering by writing only for yourself. It doesn't mean that your work is not powerful or amazing or beautiful. After all, look at Emily Dickinson, who published only ten of the nearly 2,000 poems that she wrote in her lifetime. Is she, somehow, not a poet?

Additionally, a movement out of the heart and into the mind—known to most as revision—does not mean that you will have to share your work. There is so much pleasure to be had in revising itself.

But if you want to share your work or if you want your work to be as elegant and as tight as possible, then you must climb out of your heart for the moment and reside in your head. Revision requires a different set of tools, tools that discern and remove, scrape and scrap, cleave and clear. The mind is made for the scalpel work of revision. So we ascend.

Every writer, I imagine, who has ever lived would testify to the importance of revision (okay, well, maybe not Jack Kerouac, although he did exhort us to "Believe in the holy contour of life," which at least suggests that he honored shapeliness even if he didn't revise for it). At least any writer who is being honest will testify to the power of revision. And many have done so famously. For example in *Speak, Memory*, Vladimir Nabokov writes, "I have rewritten—often several times—every word I have ever published. My pencils outlast their erasers," and Truman Capote is said to have quipped that he preferred scissors to pencils. I regularly tell my students that what separates the writers who "make it" from the writers who don't is their dedication to revision. I would suggest, if you are invested in your work reaching others, then not only must you learn to revise well but you must commit the same energy and focus to re-seeing your work as you did to birthing it. Nothing frustrates me more than a student who has their writing workshopped by the entire class, receives pages of written feedback, and spends fifteen weeks with an essay only to submit a final draft that looks almost identical to their first draft. They rearrange words like Scrabble tiles, when revision is closer to gutting a fish.

In his popular book *Writing Tools*, Roy Peter Clark offers the wise metaphor of tree trimming when he considers revision. In the first stage of shaping a tree, you lop entire limbs. In the second, you find your pruning clippers. Lopping limbs is the work of seeing the fundamental form or shape of your piece. Much is going to need to go. Lots of limbs. Big ones. You will need the chainsaw for sure. But you cannot know what to cut until you understand the deeper subject of your piece, so you cannot begin the work of revision until you have whittled your deeper subject down to that elevator pitch. A poet like Corrinne Hales might say of her poem "Power" that the poem is about two kids who play a trick on a railroad conductor, but then she might add that she is really writing about the watershed moment when we, as children, learn we can harm. Once you know your deeper subject, tape the sentence to your notebook cover or laptop or altar. It is the mantra of the piece.

You may have written twenty pages of a short story before you understood what you are really writing about. You might have created twelve scenes and three characters and a boatload of great diction that might need to be lopped once you see the fundamental shape. There is no way around this. You could not arrive where you have arrived without writing your way there. Teleporting does not exist in art. The work you needed to do to find your way toward your deeper subject has not been wasted, even if it all must be deleted. Those paragraphs, stanzas, pages, and lines did what they needed to do. They carried their load. But now they must be cut.

So cut. Cut deep and cut hard. Make yourself do it. If you cannot see the limbs to cut, then give yourself page or word limitations and enforce them. If your story is seventeen pages long, cut it down to ten. Insist on it. When we are forced to compress, our writing grows stronger. If we give ourselves fixed goals, then we have to make the decision of what cannot be excised, which means we are also making the decision of what we can afford to lose. Twenty or thirty percent of your work may remain after you lop those limbs. If you are trying to get away with something, then you delete a paragraph and hope for the best. That will never work.

One saving grace: the Mulch Folder on your desktop. In our modern world, hardly anything is ever actually gone. As you lop your limbs, copy them into your Mulch Folder. You will never know when that amazing paragraph about the mechanic who ate lunch wearing their wife's apron over their coveralls will come in handy. It didn't work for this story, but it may, yet, have another life.

Make no mistake about it. Revision is heartrending work. It's another reason that we climb out of our hearts and into our heads. The mind can wield the ax with fewer tears. I always resist revision at first. When I take my writing to my writing group, I wait for them to tell me that it is ready for *The New Yorker*, but they don't. And the moment they do tell me that my piece is perfect, I need to find a new writing group. When I move to revision, I perpetually drag my feet. In some ways, revision may appear easier because you have words in front of you and your only job is to make them better (rather than the process of birthing something out of nothing), but most writers will tell you that it is just a different kind of difficulty. When I am revising, I will insist that drafting is easier and more pleasurable. When I am drafting, I long for the moment I can revise. The grass is always greener.

Your first pass at revision, then, requires you to find your wolf and be the wolf. You must understand the fundamental shape of your work by understanding your deeper subject and then chop, gut, and chainsaw your way to that shape. Second, know that beneath every piece of writing that ever makes it into the world exist the layers and layers and layers of words that had to be written to find the right ones. The words that remain stand on top of those whose sole purpose on the page was to carve the path to clarity.

43

Collecting Language

In climbing, if there is a chance the rope could run out or, when anchoring, that the entire system could fail, you tie a catastrophe knot. To me, this says a lot about the sport. Catastrophe is possible; a knot will save your life. The same is true for the quick draws that climbers use to clip themselves to the rock face. Just like the gun slingers of the wild West, you must pull fast, before your hand slips from the rock. Routes have a crux, sometimes more than one. On a trad route, the lead climber is in charge of placing protection into the limestone or granite, and life depends on the placement. The one below who is belaying might belay through a Gri Gri, a device most likely named after an African amulet or talisman meant to ward off danger. Just like you wouldn't share underwear, most climbers I know will only belay with their own Gri Gri. Made of metal and far from cozy, the Gri Gri and climber share skin-like intimacy.

If you are not a climber, and you are writing a story about a character who is, then you might be able to name the rope, possibly the harness, the rock, though maybe not the type. If you are not a climber, then your character would climb the rock, but they might not stem, dyno, or mantle. If you are not a climber, you won't define holds as pockets or jugs or crimps. You might not even call them holds. And, I would argue, you will have lost much. A knot on its own is so commonplace that it conjures no image. A catastrophe knot, on the other hand, names the stakes and stops the reader.

The choice between knot and catastrophe knot is a choice in diction. The words we choose are all that we, as writers, have to convey our ideas. Every word, then, must be chosen with care and intention. If you are writing a story about a climber, you do not have to be a climber, but you must immerse yourself in the diction of climbing. Precise diction helps establish our authority as writers—it helps contribute to that nebulous quality of voice—and also paints a much more evocative picture for the reader. In general, when we read, we create images in our head conjured by the words.

Sometimes, in fiction and nonfiction, the images form a story; sometimes, say in poetry, the images evoke feeling more than narrative. Remember Gardner's dream. If you have any doubt as to how wed you are to the images you conjure as a reader, consider what happens when you read *Harry Potter* before you see the movie. Your Harry will be different from the movie Harry. In fact, you might reject the movie Harry at first because he looks nothing like the Harry in your head. Here's the kicker, though, once you see the movie Harry, there is a good chance the Harry in your head will be forever displaced. We are visual creatures. Our imaginings are strong but usually not as strong as what our eyes physically see. As writers, we want to lean into the physicality and materiality of language.

To state the obvious again: words are all we have to create images for our readers. That spelling and spellwork share etymologies is not happenstance. Words conjure. Words cast. In general, in English, we rely on roughly twice as many nouns as verbs and more than three times the nouns than adjectives and adverbs in our speaking and writing. Nouns, then, are the most commonly used part of speech, which is unsurprising given they name the things of the world. Nouns evoke objects, matter with weight, dimension, scale, color, and texture as well as abstractions like love, fear, anger, and hatred. Interestingly, nouns take us longer to say than verbs. Researchers have found that a speaker will pause milliseconds longer to produce a noun rather than a verb and, even more remarkable, that a listener will intuit the millisecond pause and understand that a noun is forthcoming and heighten their attention. Nouns, these linguists say, are novel. They produce more new information in communication than, say, verbs. Writing for *The New Yorker*, Alan Burdick tells us, "Verbs are grammatically more complex than nouns but have less to reveal. When you're about to say a verb, you're less likely to be saying something new, so your brain doesn't have to slow down what it's already doing to plan for it."

The author of *Call Up the Waters*, Amber Caron, spends much of her day "pulling language." Long before she even has an idea for a story, she is immersing herself in the language of whatever interests her. You only have to read her stories to see the result of such attention for they brim with the diction of oology, water witching, dog sledding, and mountain rescue. Caron says one of her favorite parts of the writing process is collecting language. Each word opens a door to a world that was previously unknown. The longer you collect language, the more precise your diction becomes: knot, to overhand knot, to catastrophe knot. Before writing her story "Calling up the Waters," a story about a water dowser, Caron spent time with *Home Ground*, a literary encyclopedia of the landscape. The book itself is a collection of sorts, offering words like "krummholz" and "loess" and "scoria" to define the landscape that surrounds us and can turn a cliff into a scarp-foot spring. Collecting words like she might eggs and gathering them all in one place led her, eventually, to water dowsing and rivers that run unseen beneath our feet.

What I appreciate about Caron's process is that it privileges language even before idea. It allows the tools themselves to do the work and assures that the writer moves from the ground up rather than from idea down. In other words, when we begin with collecting language, we begin with our feet on the earth. We begin with the things of the world, the held, the buried, the burned, the adorned, the cooked, the sunk, and the stranded. Often the advice given to writers is to make sure to get the name of the dog. A Chihuahua, say, rather than tiny brown dog. And while such precision needs to be applied in the revision process and will certainly tighten the language and create a stronger image for the reader, it is equally important to understand that diction can also lead us into our work.

Lastly, as you fill your sacks, remember that what you are gathering is not a collection of the dead and the desiccate. Language is alive. It changes and grows, transforms. It breathes. Every year, new words are added to the dictionary and the words already in our lexicon change in meaning. Queer today is not the queer of a hundred years ago. Not only does the meaning change but even its assigned part of speech. For example, one can queer a narrative or queer a classroom. It's no longer an adjective alone. Every word that we use, then, freights all past meanings, regardless of whether we are aware of them or not. We can remain ignorant (and ignorance always eventually harms) or we can be cognizant and aware of the legacy of language. In English, most of our nouns have Anglo-Saxon roots, while many of our abstractions are Latinate. Knowing this helps us understand why bowl and salt and stone have a gravity to them that a word like cerebral does not. If we are writing about something solid, certain, and heavy, we want to draw on Anglo-Saxon words. If we are writing about God, then maybe contemplation makes a better choice. On the other hand, we might use the phrase "rule of thumb" without understanding that the origin of the phrase comes from the circumference of a stick a man could legally use to beat his wife. Unintended violence would then hum beneath our poem.

Spend time tracking down the etymologies of words and phrases. Online sites like etymonline.com make the process painless, but don't forget that a good old-fashioned dictionary will teach you plenty. Open your Webster's to any page and read it like a novel. You never know when you might learn that "contemplation" (Latin) comes from the prefix "com," meaning together, and the word "templum." The templum was the hill the priest would ascend to watch the sky for birds and the messages they might bring. When Michael teaches his poetry students about etymology he always quotes Emerson, who says "words are fossil poetry." Contemplation is the word he uses as an example because it demonstrates how even Latinate words that seem abstract eventually find their way back to earth. You just have to dig.

Every word matters. At every moment in the writing process, you are making a choice to move in this direction or in that. From all possibilities available to you, you are choosing one word and, by default, not choosing all the others. When you choose a word, choose one from a bag that you have already filled. Pull your words with intention and precision. In *The Real Thing*, the playwright Tom Stoppard writes, "I don't think writers are sacred, but words are. They deserve respect. If you get the right ones in the right order, you might nudge the world a little."

44

Choosing Your Wand

In yoga, the physical world is comprised of three elements, or *tattvas*. The word *tattva* comes from *tat*, or suchness. Everything in this world, for a yogi, then has a suchness comprised of a mixture of *tamas*, *rajas*, and *sattva*, the three *gunas*. For purposes here, I will define *tamas* as a kind of dark, heavy energy, sticky, tarry, and not very fluid, while *rajas* has a kind of fiery energy, red, forceful, and very active. *Sattva* is the purest and most subtle form of energy, all upward and light-filled and even holy. Everything from a table to a tree to our mental state is comprised of the three *gunas* in varying proportions. To give a simple example, a mountain contains a lot of *tamasic* energy—heavy, fixed, ponderous. While a dog has more *rajasic* energy, panting after the squirrel in the yard. Importantly, though, the *gunas* are not static but relational. For instance, the roots of a tree contain *tamasic* qualities in the way that they cling to the earth in comparison to the leaves of the tree, which are all *sattvic* energy, reaching for the sun. That same tree, though, will be more *tamasic* when viewed in relation to the sky. So, the *gunas* are not fixed—a rock is not always *tamasic*—and everything in the physical world contains all three *gunas* but to varying degrees.

In language, verbs are what dictate the energy in a sentence, and they do so by describing the energetic relationship between the nouns. Take the sentence "The bowl sits on the table." The relationship between the bowl and the table is fairly sedentary. Not much movement, really no movement at all. The energy between the bowl and the table remains constant; a bowl sitting on a table has a good deal of *tamasic* energy, downward moving, sedate. Take another sentence, "The child walked home." The verb, once again, describes the energetic relationship between the child and home. Here, more movement, more *rajasic*. Finally, observe this sentence, "Alice considered the two choices." Here the verb, "observe," describes the relationship between Alice and the choices. In some ways, you could argue that "consider" demonstrates *tamasic* qualities because no physical action is needed, or you could argue that "consider" is more *rajasic* because it suggests an energetic back and forth, or you could decide that the verb "consider" leans more toward the third category of energy and that is *sattvic*. *Sattvic* energy is subtle energy that moves upward. In many ways, any verb that describes a relationship between the concrete and the abstract is going to invoke *sattvic* energy.

All verbs demonstrate all three energies to varying degrees and that energy will shift based on relation. My point here is to think about verbs as the energetic center for your sentences. From first grade on, we have been told that verbs are action words, but that's honestly not all that helpful. They can describe action, but they can just as easily describe inaction or abstraction. When we think of verbs as determining the energetic relationships between the nouns, we see their power to bind and describe but also their ability to direct. In general, whether working with water, electricity, or language, we want to channel the energy to make it useful. Verbs channel.

In English, many of our verbs derive from Anglo-Saxon roots. Think of the lives of the early Anglos, not a lot of time for deep contemplation. Instead, they spent their days hunting, growing, fighting, and trying to stay alive. They bequeathed a legacy of muscular verbs that populate our writing and speech. These verbs are not fancy thesaurus verbs; they tend to be more meat-and-potatoes verbs. They will be the verbs you reach for most often.

Below is a paragraph from Anthony Doerr's novel *Cloud Cuckoo Land*. I have underlined the main verb in each sentence.

> He <u>escorts</u> five fifth graders from the elementary school to the public library through curtains of falling snow. He <u>is</u> an octogenarian in a canvas coat; his boots <u>are fastened</u> with Velcro; cartoon penguins <u>skate</u> across his necktie. All day, joy <u>has</u> steadily <u>inflated</u> inside his chest, and now, this afternoon, at 4:30 p.m. on a Thursday in February, watching the children run ahead down the sidewalk—Alex Hess wearing his papier-mâché donkey head, Rachel Wilson carrying a plastic torch, Natalie Hernandez lugging a portable speaker—the feeling <u>threatens</u> to capsize him.

Let's begin where Doerr does: with "escort." Not Anglo-Saxon but rather Latinate. What is the energetic relationship between Zeno (the he) and the fifth graders? Escort certainly has *rajasic* movement, but it is a guided movement. Escort suggests an element of care, like that of a teacher. Doerr could have said something like "he leads," but Doerr reached for a verb with more *sattvic* energy (upward moving, intellectual), so he chose "escort" and its underlying connection to protection. His verb is describing the energetic relationship that Zeno has with the fifth graders. He is not dictator demanding obedience; he is walking alongside.

For the moment, we will skip the second verb ("is") and move to boots that are fastened and penguins that skate. "Fasten" is Anglo-Saxon in origin and suggests a fairly *tamasic* relationship between the boots and the Velcro. Nothing is moving. While the origins of "skate" are a bit harder to trace, they appear to be early German and suggest movement. The movement is ironic, though, because the penguins remain fixed on the tie. Notice the energy being channeled by Doerr's verb choice in that sentence—the energy is both fixed and moving. Zeno is an old man, in his eighties we learn in the second sentence, but Doerr, through his verbs, is letting the reader know that while his body has slowed, he has not.

Now consider the final sentence where joy (an abstract quality) "has ... inflated" throughout the day. The verb "inflate" is Latinate, describing the energy of joy as it moves in his body (all *sattvic*, upward, subtle). The verb moves up, the joy moves up, the energy moves up until (after the long embrace of a parenthetical) we arrive at the second subject, "feeling," which relates back to joy, and we discover that the feeling "threatens to capsize." "Threat" is Anglo-Saxon and has a kind of ax-solid solidity to it. The feeling of joy—all upward moving, Latinate, abstract, *sattvic*—threatens to capsize him, taking us back down to the ground and planting the seeds in the savvy reader's mind that this joy will bring Zeno sorrow.

The opening paragraph to Zeno's story: pure magic.

Did Doerr pay attention to each and every verb? Yes. Especially if you read Doerr's work, you will understand how intentionally Doerr cultivates his verbs. Did Doerr consider whether each verb he chose was Latinate or Low German or Dutch in origin as he revised? Probably not. But does Doerr know, intuitively, as a human born to write and who, therefore, must write, who has dedicated his life to words and the spell they cast, who spends whole days immersed in the sea of language, that verbs channel energy? For sure.

The lesson here is one of paying attention and understanding that verbs describe the energetic relationship between the words in the sentence. You never need to reach for a thesaurus. None of the verbs that Doerr chooses in the above paragraph are fancy by any means. They are intentional. And they channel the movement of the lines—even when, and maybe especially when, the movement is less than linear (to both fasten and skate). Like significant detail, the verbs that Doerr has selected work on two levels. Readers won't see that at first, but Doerr is already hinting at what will lead to Zeno's death: love. His joy will capsize his body.

Choose your verbs with care. Understand that they are designating energy. A paragraph populated by forms of the verb "to be" is a paragraph that gives the reader almost no understanding of the energetic relationship between the nouns. Compare something as simple as "The bowl sits on the table" versus "The bowl is on the table." On a literal level, the two sentences say the same thing. Both tell the reader the location of the bowl. But even the little bit of energy invoked by "sit" will generate a stronger image in the reader's head about the relationship between the bowl and the table. "Sit" is a tiny bit more evocative and gives the reader the hint of rest and ease that "is" does not. In general, you want to remove almost every linking verb from your work (forms of to be, as well as appear, seem, even feel). Those verbs are empty of energetic description. They rarely channel or direct.

That said, a form of "to be" does have a place to shine in our sentences and that's when it is doing exactly what it is meant to do: show equality—a kind of static energy—two wands dueling and neither giving way. When "to be" is used with such intention, then what would first appear to be empty of energy becomes more charged. Consider the second sentence in Doerr's paragraph: "He is an octogenarian." At first glance, it could appear like that sentence has lost its energetic center—not unlike "The bowl is on the table." But if you think of "is" here as the equal sign, as it is meant to be syntactically, then all of a sudden Zeno and octogenarian become the same thing—they are charged to each other. And because Doerr selects "octogenarian" rather than eighty-year-old, we understand, as readers, that Zeno remains far from infirm. He claims his age and the wisdom that has come from living on the earth for close to a century. "He is an octogenarian," then, becomes filled with power. He might as well be Superman.

If a reader tells you that your prose is flat or that your poem is cerebral, you want to turn to your verbs. As the energetic element in language, verbs create movement. They channel and direct, even when that direction creates opposition. Even when a character is stuck or a poem is pursuing the abstract, or the narrator is mired in depression and cannot make their way out of bed, the language cannot be devoid of movement. Your verbs can invoke the loss of energy but they, themselves, must channel that loss. When describing the most delicate of events, a crocus unfolding at first sun, your verbs need to be muscular and strong. As you move to the finer points of revision, underline every verb in your poem, story, or essay. Earn the linking verbs that you allow to remain; burn the rest. And then find the verb that carries the energy needed in each sentence. Ultimately, the current runs from first word to last, born by the verbs, unblocked and unfettered.

45

Heart Holding

Almost a month ago to the day I am writing, the Buddhist monk Thich Nhat Hanh left his body as well as a legacy of kindness. Thay, as his devotees called him, was a Vietnamese peace activist who founded Plum Village, helped bring mindfulness to the West, and wrote more than a hundred books on the practice. Known as the father of mindfulness, his passing was mourned by millions, though his presence will remain with even more. Thich Nhat Hanh offered several breathing practices that combined the breath and the heart. The one I outline below is just an introduction to the gifts he has given the world.

For this heart-holding practice, you simply begin, once again, in a comfortable seated pose. Find your three-part breath, nourishing your lungs and body. When you are ready, turn to your four- and six-count breath, feeling mind and body settle with the long exhalation. Everything slows down. Allow your exhalation to carve deeper channels; encourage the inhalation to fill to your edges. At this point, the breath is only miracle. Fullness, to emptiness, to fullness. Breathe here for a few minutes.

Now take your left hand to your heart and your right hand to cover your left. Honestly, this act alone will often make me cry. When I hold my heart, I become simultaneously aware of my own mortality and fragility as well as how loved I am. People in my life, Michael, Aidan, Kellen, my parents, friends, all come before my closed eyes the moment I place the palms of my hands to my heart space. If you are quiet enough, you can feel the beat of your heart, perhaps even feel the pulse echo in your throat or ears. Keep breathing. Notice that every inhalation passes through the gate of the heart, and every exhalation takes the same path on its way to void. The heart is the transom or threshold for the breath as well as the location of the fourth chakra.

In yoga, there are multiple chakra systems, but in the West we generally think of seven chakras that energetically run the length of the spine from coccyx to crown of the head. Briefly, we begin at the base of the spine with the root chakra, *mūlādhāra*. Embodying the earth element, this chakra provides our sense of groundedness and stability and relates to basic needs like food and water. The second chakra, *svādhisthāna*, is the abode of emotion and sexuality. Mirroring our emotional landscape, the second chakra is related to the element of water. The third chakra, *manipūra*, is located at our solar plexus and is home to the element of fire. Our worldly power is found in this chakra, as well as what Kabir calls our "wanting creature." The fourth chakra, *anāhata*, and the one I focus on below, is at the heart and corresponds with the element of air. Love, like air, has no boundaries. At the base of our throat is the *viśuddha* chakra. You can think of this chakra as the place for intuition or deeper perception. Its element is ether, the space between the atoms. Both the sixth chakra, *ājñā*, our third eye, and the seventh chakra, *sahasrāra*, hovering just above the crown of the head, are considered beyond language. It is thought that in yoga when spiritual energy rises to the sixth and seventh chakra you have an enlightenment experience—a moment of seeing the connection between everything, oneness. In their upward movement from the dense to the subtle, at the most basic level, the chakras remind us that we contain all.

The heart chakra serves as the middle chakra in this system, connecting the lower three chakras, which are generally concerned with matters of this world, with the upper three chakras, which are generally concerned with the unmanifest or divine. The heart occupies the middle space, and in Tantra is represented by two intersecting triangles, one pointing up and the other pointing down. You can find lots of books that describe how to activate or envision these energy centers, and certainly my purpose here is not to explore the subtle body but I find the image of two intersecting triangles informative in terms of why our heart matters to us so much (aside from, of course, its physical necessity). The first triangle points downward and focuses us on our loved ones, whether those are human, nonhuman, or arboreal. Love forms the underlying nature of everything in the world. Love compels us, sustains us, challenges us, and brings suffering. Beneath every emotion, every experience, resides love, even something as simple as opening the door and seeing a billowy white cloud in the shape of an angelfish swim by. So the downward pointing triangle represents our everyday experience of love on this planet. We know what love feels like. That's why we sorrow.

The upward pointing triangle directs us toward a higher kind of love, a love without limits or conditions, a kind of love rarely achieved by humans. But a love we have tasted. We all have had those flashes when we feel the boundaries of our individual self give way to a larger self, one without boundaries. Maybe it is when we stand before a sunset or a painting or hear a piece of music that makes us cry. Maybe it is when our first child arrives in the world or our mother slips from it while holding our hand. Some people call this larger sense of connection God, but you don't need to name it. Just feel it. In those moments of pure peace, pure grace, pure joy, we touch this larger love. In yoga, that love is called *prema*. It's a love that never begins, ends, or diminishes. It is through the heart that we are led downward toward the love we feel for each other and then upward toward a love that cannot be named.

That is how the heart becomes the gate, and that is why holding the heart can immediately make us weep. We are touching the entrance to the vertical while standing on the horizontal.

Hold your heart and breathe. Then, on your next inhalation, say, "Breathing in, I feel my heart." On your exhalation, say silently, "Breathing out, I smile." And as you breathe out, turn the corners of your mouth to the sky and feel your heart illumine. That's all. A simple practice that brings equanimity.

Thich Nhat Hanh taught that "our own life has to be our message." I love the idea that we write with our lives first and then with our pens. In this meditation, he encourages us to see smiling as peace work and to notice how the smile is the source or joy rather than joy needing to happen before the smile. We build our happiness like we build our sentences. A smile, like a word, is the start. Breathe with a sweet smile on your face for as long as it feels good, and then open your eyes and be the message.

46

Word by Word by Word

When all those really concrete nouns come together with all those energetic verbs and are further adorned by articles, prepositions, pronouns, and so on, sentences are born. A collection of words and phrases assembled in an arrangement, whether pleasing or not, is called syntax. Generally speaking, writers revise toward syntax that is euphonious to the ear, expressed in the fewest words possible, illuminates deeper subject, and creates texture on the page. At the end of revision, you direct your attention to each and every sentence, and you consider how that sentence is working as a syntactical unit as well as how it relates to the other sentences around it. This sounds more technical than it is. Most writers rely largely on their ear to "hear" how the syntax is working. The more you write, the more attuned your ear becomes. But there are some basic principles that you can keep in mind as you read your prose or poem for syntax, when you revise for style. At this point, you have cut the limbs, tended the nouns and verbs, and now you are down in the weeds of your lines. The most compelling characters in the world will never come to life in a reader's head if the reader keeps stumbling on the syntax.

First, pay attention to your sentence variety. Basically, you want it and probably don't have it. In the Western world, we tend to cultivate right-branching sentences. Read the newspaper, and you will be convinced. A right-branching sentence looks like this sentence. It begins with the subject, followed directly by the verb. So, "sentence" is my subject and "looks" is my very weak verb. The reason Western readers prefer right-branching sentences is that the information needed to make meaning is delivered right away. We, as readers, know who is doing what. It grounds us. We like that. In fact, once we have the subject and the verb, we, as readers, are willing to let the writer tack on as many clauses and descriptors as they want following the subject and verb. As writers, we want to write into that preference, meaning, most of our sentences will begin with the subject closely followed by the verb. Or at least a lot of them will. But if every sentence begins subject then verb, the syntax becomes anything but pleasing. The writing feels flat, boring, and dull. We might describe it as "bad" writing, though we might not know what makes it "bad."

So we need variety. Some sentences, maybe many, will begin subject followed by verb, but then some might begin with several clauses stacked in a series, before the subject is ever named. Withholding the subject or main verb creates a kind of mini-tension for the reader. The writer makes the choice to delay the subject or verb because they want the reader to feel a little uneasy, a little lost, a little confused. In that way, syntax underscores deeper meaning but on a sentence level. We will look at an example below.

Another way to revise with sentence variety in mind is to count the number of words in every sentence. You may find that you generally write eleven-word sentences. Sentences that are similar in length can also begin to feel tedious. Sometimes you want to pull the reader up short by slamming them with a three-word fragment. Punch them in the gut syntactically at the same time, say, your character is being metaphorically knocked down. You want to take care not to overuse such a move. If every paragraph ends on a snappy fragment, you are punching no one. Instead, a writerly tic.

Your syntax becomes stronger when you pay attention to the sonorous qualities of language—how language sounds. This is the bread and butter of poetry. Even when we don't hear a sentence out loud, in other words, when we are just reading words on the page, we intuit the harmony of the lines. The words "sound" in our heads, even if they do not pass our lips. Syntax, like all writing, is a made thing. It doesn't drop down out of the sky fully realized. We build it. And we often build it with intention. So, for example, we consider our choice in an adjective based on its resonances with the noun the adjective will modify. And those resonances are created by assonance and consonance as well as alliteration. Assonance is the way the vowels in words hook together; consonance is the way consonants bind in a word or between words; and alliteration is when words are united by the same first letter. We can also pay attention to the actual sound of the letters and their effect—for example, the word "buzz" sounds like the noise a bee makes.

What does this look like in practice? For an example, we will look at Peggy Shumaker's short essay entitled "Moving Water, Tucson." Shumaker is a poet by training, and honestly it's to the poets we should look when thinking about sonic qualities of language and concision in syntax. Of all the writers, poets work in the tightest spaces, so each word must do more than simply one thing. Many writers I know begin their day with poetry because it primes their own pumps of language. A poet like Audre Lorde gives us the first line from her poem "Coal"

> I
> Is the total black, being spoken
> From the earth's inside.

and we could spend the rest of our day just sitting with that image.

As a poet, Shumaker hooks her words together and revises to underscore meaning. Consider the first sentences of her essay: "Thunderclouds gathered every afternoon during the monsoons. Warm rain felt good on faces lifted to lick water from the sky. We played outside, having sense enough to go out and revel in the rain. We savored the first cool hours since summer hit." Notice, first, that all of these sentences are right-branching. They begin, very directly, subject and verb. Shumaker is establishing a pattern, a rhythm in her syntax that she will soon disrupt. For the moment, though, she wants the reader to feel the certainty of being grounded in the minutes before a flash flood arrives. Her syntax helps to instill the feeling of stability.

Notice, though, that while her sentences arrive fairly uniform in length and follow a deliberate subject-verb pattern, the words within the sentences have strong sonic qualities. In the first sentence, the "th" of thunderclouds hooks into the "th" of gathered. And the "oo" on afternoon binds that word to the "oo" in monsoon. Her sentences are tight and connected at the start of the essay, just like the world before the flash flood. Any rain, here, is a delight in a desert landscape where, she writes later, "water is always holy." We can also see her play with the sonorous qualities of language with the words "savored" and "since" and "summer" all sizzling like hot pavement. Alliteration harmonizes the second sentences where she describes faces "lifted to lick" and then later they "revel in the rain." Syntax at the start of the essay is all about welding words to one another and grounding the reader through right-branching prose.

By the second paragraph, the flood has begun with "moving water" that begins to fill the arroyo. It starts to lift debris in its rush. Here, Shumaker turns from the solidity of right-branching syntax to the shards of sentence fragments. "Tumbleweed, spears of ocotillo, creosote, a doll's arm, some kid's fort." And then, "Broken bottles, a red sweater." All the items being picked up in the growing flood. The fragments have power *because* we were given right-branching, uniform sentences first. A rhythm was established and then broken, broken at the very moment the banks of the arroyo give way.

By the fourth paragraph, a kid steps forth from the collective "we" that has been narrating the piece. He actually doesn't step forth but rather steps into the flood and tries to ride the flash on a piece of plywood. When the water takes him down, transfigures him from hero to horror, Shumaker unleashes a run-on sentence that gushes the length of eight lines. The sentence is the only left-branching sentence in the essay. Water and land come at us, "trees, root wads and all," clause after clause after clause. We can't breathe. The syntax won't let us. We gulp for air. Then we arrive at the subject and the verb, "we couldn't step back."

It goes without saying that her run-on sentence, the way it drowns the reader as it drowns the kid in the flood, could only have such an effect because Shumaker began with right-branching sentences, moved to fragments, and then let her line unravel. I would argue that her syntax is doing as much, even more, than the actual setting, the physical tension, or the interesting choice in point of view. When we revise, we want to pay this kind of attention to our syntax. Language casts a spell. It transmutes the unseen into the seen. You want your spell to be a powerful one, one filled with intention. Of spell casting in general, Pam Grossman says, "Knowing just the right combination of syllables can unlock a secret door or manifest a desired outcome." Shumaker deprives her reader of breath; she makes them gasp for air like the kid whose life is about to be lost. And she does this with words.

One final suggestion. Read your work out loud. Many times. Many times. Many times. Shut the door to your room and read. Don't whisper. Don't read in your head. It's not the same. Read your work in a clear, strong voice. We want our language to sing. For that to happen, it must move like a song. When you read your work out loud, you will hear the places where you stumble or the places where the syntax is flat and boring. Attend to those places. If you falter when you read, you might want to cast a better spell.

47

Taking Refuge

In Buddhism, a practitioner can formalize their commitment to the path through a ritual that is called taking refuge. Once you decide that you want to be a Buddhist, you would, formally or informally, vow to take refuge in the three jewels: the Buddha, the *dharma*, and the *sangha*, thereby signaling your dedication. The first of the three jewels, the Buddha himself, becomes the example you follow, and the *dharma*, which are the teachings, create a kind of path. The third jewel or support, the *sangha*, contains all beings who have made similar vows. They form your fellowship. The revered Buddhist monk Chögyam Trungpa Rinpoche elaborates, "By taking this particular vow, we end our shopping in the spiritual supermarket. We decide to stick to a particular brand for the rest of our lives. We choose to stick to a particular staple diet and flourish on it." In his words, especially the commitment to a single way of finding meaning and truth, I see many similarities with our own commitments to writing: that one becomes a writer because one must. Born to write, we no longer consider a degree in interior design or buying a potter's wheel. We choose to write because writing chose us. Writers share many similarities with yogis and Buddhists, with anyone who dedicates their lives to the search for meaning through one-pointed focus and attention. You made a very similar vow when you decided to claim the robes of writer without any need for external reward or affirmation. You make the vow anew every morning that you show up to write.

Chögyam Trungpa Rinpoche continues to explain how taking refuge is anything other than scurrying back to your mother's arms in hopes that she will save you. He says, "We have to work with the sense of sacredness and richness and the magical aspect of our experience. And this has to be done on the level of our everyday existence, which is a personal level, an extremely personal level. There are no scapegoats. When you take refuge you become responsible to yourself." In other words, like Rilke, he insists that we cannot look outside of ourselves for someone to tell us what to do. Not our parents, not our partners, not our teachers, not our editors, not our readers. When we commit, truly commit, to any practice, whether writing or dancing or meditating, our faith is in the work alone.

And a path that you enter by taking responsibility for yourself can feel very lonely. As children, we ran to our mother's (or any safe caregiver's) arms because she affirmed our worthiness by telling us she loved us; she affirmed our rightness by saying we had done nothing wrong; she affirmed our place by calling us hers. It was pretty nice. The etymology of refuge comes from *re* (to return) and *fugio* (to flee), so basically a refuge is the place we flee back to. And when times are hard, the place most of us want to flee to is our best version of home and the person tending the hearth at the center. Not unlike the vow to Buddhism, a commitment to writing requires that we step into our own power, which simultaneously means giving none of our power away by blaming others or asking to be saved. When Chögyam Trungpa Rinpoche writes of taking refuge in Buddhism, he says, "You commit yourself as a refugee to yourself, no longer thinking that some divine principle that exists in the holy law or holy scriptures is going to save you. It is very personal. You experience a sense of loneliness, aloneness—a sense that there is no savior, no help."

But, he continues, that doesn't mean you are outside companionship. The third support to aid a practicing Buddhist is the *sangha*. In yoga, we use the word *satsang*, which means a group (*sangha*) of truth (*sat*) seekers. The *satsang* are your companions on the path. It's a kind of independent togetherness. Chögyam Trungpa Rinpoche writes, "But at the same time there is a sense of belonging: you belong to a tradition of loneliness where people work together." The *satsang* doesn't exist to reassure you. It doesn't exist to tell you what you need to do or be. "Instead," Chögyam Trungpa Rinpoche writes, "each member of the *sangha* is an individual who is on the path in a different way from all the others. It is because of that that you get constant feedback of all kinds: negative and positive, encouraging and discouraging."

As a writer who is born to write, you need a *satsang*, a group of truth seekers who are able to walk their own path without needing anyone to tell them where that path lies. Some people call this a writing group. I like *satsang* because it puts the emphasis on the fact that everyone in the group is seeking and what they are seeking is truth. A writing group, then, is a group of people who have made the commitment to externalize that which is internal, to name their truth through language.

While you must walk your own path (and will suffer greatly if you try and walk someone else's), you do not walk it alone. You have to find your kindred spirits. No one can really tell you where they reside. They may live in groups formed at the library or a bookstore or by a humanities or arts council or a league of writers; they may be found online or at yoga class or at church; they might attend a class or workshop that you have taken; they might appear as a Facebook group or a note pinned to a bulletin board at the coffee shop down the street. Most likely, you will need to build your *satsang*. If you are looking for someone else to do it for you, then you have not made a vow to the writing life. A writing group can simply consist of two people who agree to share work every week. A writing group might gather twenty people together who live in the same town and meet every Tuesday at the library for cold reads. It doesn't matter how many companions form your *satsang*, whether they are famous, well read, or well published. In many ways, it works better if everyone stands on the same ground. Your companions just have to be seeking the truth in ways that you recognize and trust.

My writing group currently consists of five people. We meet monthly at each other's houses and share physical drafts. My friend Rona has a writing group that meets online every week and requires that each person produce a certain number of pages that they don't actually share. Instead they spend their time talking about the writing and their process. A class will offer you a formal writing group that might consist of the entire class or a smaller section of the class. Again, it doesn't matter. It only matters that you find like-minded people who are working at a similar pace and are willing to meet as often as you would like to meet.

In writing, we basically have two places to take refuge, two jewels. The first is in the work itself and the second is with fellow writers. Those refuges will not always feel happy and warm and familiar. Sometimes, often, the work of writing feels less like refuge and more like torture chamber. And sometimes our writing group, our *satsang*, offers feedback that feels disappointing or overwhelming. As Trungpa writes, the *satsang* is there to serve as a mirror. Everyone in the *satsang* is seeking truth (externalizing their internal truth), but each on their own path. We look to our companions to let us know how we are doing. And, Chögyam Trungpa Rinpoche says, that means they will support us with feedback that tells us where we are doing well as when we are falling short. It is hard to take criticism. Believe me, I know. Remember, even after three decades, I arrive at my writing group hoping they will crown me Queen of the Essay. But we need those mirrors. They are all we have in determining whether what we have cast comes close to what we experienced on the inside. O'Keeffe writes Stieglitz about her latest work: "I ask because I wonder if I got over to anyone what I want to say." Stieglitz is her *satsang*, her companion, her mirror.

Two final points. Finding your writing group is like finding a good therapist: the fit must be there. The last thing in the world that you need as you dedicate yourself day in and day out to the page would be for others to meet your work with hostility, jealously, and meanness. In my experience with thousands upon thousands of pages of student writing, a reader can meet a draft of a poem or story from one of two positions: either looking for ways to find fault or assuming the best at every turn. You want to find the generous readers, for they will most likely also be able to deliver criticism in a way that you can hear. Find a writing group in which you can take refuge, not because they hold your hand and tell you that you are Walt

Whitman reincarnated but rather because the mirror they hold allows you to see your own work with love and tenderness. Their feedback opens the door to revision, rather than slamming the door shut to ever writing again.

Second, determine the shape of the feedback that you would like to receive. The current conversation surrounding writing workshops and feedback is focused on assuring that the writer remains in charge of the process so that they retain their agency and power. Sharing your work with others is always hard and scary. To feel like your role is to simply sit quietly while the rest of the group decides what it is you are trying to say can reinscribe feelings of powerlessness and even abuse that you have experienced in your life. The work is yours, and you are in charge of deciding what is most useful to you in terms of feedback. Based on the work of Felicia Rose Chavez and her book *The Anti-Racist Writing Workshop*, I would suggest writing a letter to your group every time it is your turn to share your work. The letter would begin by stating, in one or two sentences, what your work is about— what your artistic vision is. While the letter might then reflect on process or describe challenges, it would end with three craft-based questions to guide the discussion. For example, you might describe your concern that one of your characters feels like a stereotype or maybe you worry that the form is too gimmicky. Because you have already stated your intention as a writer, those responding can consider the work in relation to your intent—rather than more generally in terms of whether they "like" it. Such a letter pulls double duty. In writing the letter, you must articulate your artistic vision and it guides your companions in considering how to help you realize that intention.

Do you have to have a writing group? No, not at all. You can decide to dedicate yourself to the process alone and know that the act of writing every day is opening both your mind and heart. But a *satsang* can be a powerful part of your practice. Remember, for a Buddhist, the strength of companions on the path turns out to be as central a support to the vow as the Buddha himself. Companion writers walk a similar path; they know it can be dark and lonely; they understand as well how the work satisfies, how it fills, how it nourishes. They, too, are born to write. They, too, face a blank page every day. And that's why they will be the very first ones to encourage, to light a candle, to hold the mirror with care, and to remind you that your only job is to write. You let the rest go.

48

The Public in Publication

Michael is friends with fellow-Utah poet Katharine Coles. An accomplished poet with several books of poetry as well as awards from the National Endowment for the Arts and the National Science Foundation, Coles embodies for many what it means to be a writer. One day, Michael and Katie were talking about the state of poetry and how few Americans read contemporary poetry. As is common for writers, they eventually found themselves on the subject of publication and how difficult it can be to place poems in top literary journals as well as whether those poems are even read. Michael turned to Katie and said, "It's frustrating to have so few readers."

If you write long enough, you will probably express a similar concern. Maybe it will arrive in the form of a question: What's the point? While the process of writing itself can and will sustain, as soon as you move to the possibility of audience, the value of your work can feel diminished. We only ask, "What's the point?" when we have moved away from writing for the sake of writing and toward writing for an audience. You don't have to entertain enormous publication dreams to want your work to have an effect. The simple act of asking a partner or friend to read your story or essay automatically lifts your head from the page and causes you to wonder if anyone cares. When it feels like no one cares, either because they respond with confusion rather than praise or because a literary journal rejects your work, it hurts. Face enough confusion, rejection, and exclusion, and you start to wonder what's the point.

Let me return to the conversation between Michael and Katie. When Michael said, "It's frustrating to have so few readers," Katie responded, "How many is enough?" Such a good question. Do you need ten people to have read your poem? A hundred? Thousands? Tens of thousands? Millions? I can imagine you asking yourself this question and actually coming up with an answer. At this moment, 2,000 readers would be great! But here's the problem. That number will increase. You may begin by finding warmth in the knowledge that your family has read and loves your work, but then you begin to want more. You set your sights on a few poems published in a local collection. And for a moment, that satisfies. But then you think about chapbook contests and you submit to fifty of those and then win. The day the email arrives, you begin to question whether that particular contest was actually "good enough." Maybe the press was too regional, too narrow, too political, too boring. A full-length collection, you tell yourself, is all that you need. Press run of 500. No, press run of 1,000. And that happens. But no one seems to notice. Your book wins no awards. If it wins no awards, you think, then it must not be very good. You need a second collection, a better press, a better publicist, or a website. Then you will finally have arrived. People will know your work. They will be changed by it.

You see how it goes. And it goes like this for *every* writer I have ever met. Even as we shake our heads and reaffirm to one another that it's the work that matters, the moment we begin to seek an audience is the moment we begin to find lack in our ability, our art, the very belief that we were born to write.

I remember once, years ago, riding in an elevator in Angell Hall at the University of Michigan. A fiction writer from the faculty had recently appeared on the cover of *Poets & Writers*, and the poets in the elevator, who shall remain nameless, were complaining that they had not yet graced the cover of a magazine that appears six times a year. Two poets, in an elevator in Ann Arbor, complaining that they had not yet been one of the six faces in a year to appear on a publication that serves writers from around the world. Holy crow.

But their desire to appear on the cover is honestly no different than your desire for your parents to like your story. It comes from the same space: seeking external validation for your worth as a writer. We may cast aspersions on the two Michigan poets, call them whiners, name their arrogance, but they have just moved deeper into the well of wanting than you have. Wanting is wanting is wanting is wanting.

When Katie asked Michael, "How many is enough?" she was pointing out the slipperiness of the slope. You think fifty is enough, but then, one day, you are bemoaning the fact that you were only nominated for the National Book Award and didn't actually win it. One way to answer Katie is to say that no number is enough. And, in practice, for most writers, that is indeed the case. Many writers, many humans, are swimming in their wanting wells, exhausted from the efforts to stay afloat but unable to climb the mossy sides. Another answer to Katie's question is that one is enough. What if, by some incredible grace or stroke of luck, you were able to cast a spell of language that gave form to the not-yet-born that exists inside you well enough that another human being, swirling in their own experience of being human, recognized the truth of your expression because it resembled theirs or radicalized theirs or challenged theirs or altered theirs and they then rejoiced. Or maybe they cried. Or turned angry. Or maybe they held it dear because for the first time they recognized their own longing to be understood and they found that recognition in the words that you made. Maybe they never tell you that. Maybe they never meet you or know you. Maybe you never know that they have been moved. But they have been. They have been changed because of something you wrote. And they now carry your efforts inside their bodies. What a miracle if this could happen just once. Just once.

You will never know, for the most part, if or how your words are carried in the hearts of other human beings. Sure, a reader might come up to you after a reading and say something or someone might write you an email or even a letter. But in general, you won't know. Which means that the question of audience is not unlike the question of whether to write in the first place. You must have faith. And faith, by definition, cannot be proven by numbers or book sales or awards given out by foundations. One reader is all that matters, and you may never meet that reader. Faith.

Finally, before you begin the process of formal publication, you might consider alternative ways for making your work public. Here in Logan, we have a local open-mic night held twice a month called Helicon West. Writers from all over the valley attend, and the writing runs the gamut. "Well-published" and award-winning writers stand up and read their work, followed by a high school student or stay-at-home mom or someone like Ron, a man who reads two poems at every open-mic. Ron has an intellectual disability; his poems arrive just above a whisper, jumbled words without spaces in between, tumbling from lips that hardly move. Always in rhymed couplets, the poems often explore love or God, but not in ways we would initially call art. For example, he begins a poem by wondering what kind of day it will be. He writes, "Will it be a day where you just have fun? / Or will it be a day when you get things done." Another commences with the speaker confessing, "Brenan I miss you. I can't believe you're gone." That poem concludes, "Now I have to say good bye to you / Until we meet again in the next life too." The poems are simple, even simplistic, but they reveal fundamental human desires we all recognize. More importantly, they are offered by a human being who was born to write, even if many would say he has trouble even speaking. I carry Ron's poems with me, and I am humbled by his dedication and bravery.

Check and see what local opportunities exist for you to share your work. Libraries and coffee houses provide good places to begin. If an open mic doesn't exist, maybe you can look into starting one. I know of writers who host readings in their back yards and living rooms. You can also work with other local writers and create DIY zines that can be sold or left, guerilla-style, on random grocery store shelves or bus seats. Leave your work for another, an even greater gift because it is unexpected. Remember, just one reader. Anything else is missing the point.

49

Rejection as Protection

I remember, as if it were yesterday, the moment when my first child, Aidan, outgrew newborn Pampers. He was six weeks. At the time, newborn Pampers came in a lemon-yellow box, and the waistband was fuzzed like the hair on Aidan's head. Blue elephants and purple giraffes ambled from one hip to the other. I cried. When Michael came in to ask me what was wrong, I said, "He will never be a newborn again."

Dramatic, yet what I felt. Even though Aidan had only been outside the womb for six weeks, it felt like the first moment in a long series of moments that we call parenting where he was moving away from us. Nothing in my life has been as bittersweet as watching Aidan and Kellen in their becoming. We have neared the point where both will be in college, and the house, measurably quieter. Friends reassure me that they will eventually return but without the teenage angst. Still, I would give so much to start the whole journey again. I never want them to leave; I am so proud of them as they do. Bittersweet.

When we make the choice to send our work out to literary journals, or contests, presses, or agents, we have decided, then, to send our heart into the world. It's not unlike leaving your child for the first day of kindergarten. Pain and joy will follow in equal amounts. You surrender control the moment you hit the submit button. The work must stand on its own, and there is every chance in the world that it will be rejected. But we make the decision to send our work out for the same reason we leave our kids at kindergarten. The work is ready, and we want it to live outside our hearts.

No one can tell you when your poem or story is finished. Many writers say that work is never finished; revisions can always be made. In what I write here, I can only give you some guidelines. The market and the process change so quickly that anything I committed to print would be outdated within a year. I offer some practical advice that has served me well as a way to approach submitting. But like every other moment in the writing process, the labor of placing your work falls to you. Students constantly ask me where to submit their writing. And I rarely give them specific answers because I understand, from practice, that you are the only one who can find the right home for your poem. You must do the research, familiarize yourself with the field, know the journals and the contests. There are no shortcuts here either. Just as you wouldn't leave your five-year-old at the door of just any old classroom, you don't want to send your work out without knowing that the fit is there, the time is right, and that your aesthetic aligns with that of the journal/contest/agent that you are querying. The more work you do *before* you submit your work, the better chance you have in placing it.

It goes without saying that you only send out your best work, work that has been thoroughly revised, work that has been read and critiqued by your writing group, work that you know so well you can almost recite lines and paragraphs in your head. Once your work is ready, then literary journals are a good place to begin. For the most part, literary journals are small publications, online and print, that are typically housed at colleges and universities and often associated with MFA or creative PhD programs. As a beginning writer, it makes sense to look for literary journals open to new writers, as well as journals that narrow the pool of those who can submit. Some literary journals only take work from undergraduates or only veterans or only those who live with mental illness. Anything that helps to winnow down the numbers of writers who are eligible will, of course, give your work a better chance. The top literary journals receive 4,000 or 5,000 submissions *every month*. If they publish six issues, each containing three stories, three essays, and twenty poems, well, you see why rejection is the most likely outcome. The odds are never in your favor. Yet ....

You press on. Websites like newpages.com and pw.org offer incredible databases that can expose you to journals you previously did not know. The filters on these websites allow you to select for genre or for cost or for contests only. Your local library may subscribe to literary journals, or you can find literary journals for sale at bookstores and coffee shops. Online literary journals are often free and require no subscription to access. Finally, most literary journals will post some of the work they publish on their websites, even if they are print-based journals. And you will want to familiarize yourself with as many literary journals as you can because each literary journal has what is called a footprint. No two journals are alike. And it's up to you to figure out what the aesthetic of each journal is. For example, do they tend toward linear or nonlinear work? Do they like language poetry or narrative poetry? Do they want work from southern writers only? Do they have a commitment to the environment? The arts? Social justice? Multimodality? It is your job, as a writer, to find out. No one can tell you. You have to do the leg work.

It doesn't make sense for a language poet to send their work to a journal that regularly publishes long, narrative work, and it doesn't make sense for a writer with a story about childhood and illness to send to a magazine with a commitment to stories of war. There are journals out there that will never accept my work because the work I tend to write is not the work they like to publish. The fit is not there. It doesn't matter how strong my writing is, those editors will never take it. And it is a waste of everyone's time for me to send to any journal without understanding the footprint of that journal. Most journals take six months to a year to respond to writers (see above: 4,000 submissions a month), so you spend a lot of time waiting. If you haven't done your homework and have sent to a place with poor fit, then those months of waiting are fairly senseless. Do your research.

I encourage writers to start at the bottom and work up. Perhaps that is because I am an old-school writer who believes that writing is a craft in which you apprentice, so you must pay your dues. Start with journals that welcome new writers. For the most part, you will never have heard of the journal before. If it is housed in a university, then you can trust that it is a solid place for your work. My students tend to know maybe three places to publish, *The New Yorker*, *Harper's*, and *The Atlantic*. Not only might that be impossible—for example, *Harper's* only accepts unsolicited fiction—but it makes no sense. You build your reputation and status as a writer one publication at a time. Think fire. Start small.

When ready, send your poems, essay, or story to five or six different journals at one time. Almost every journal allows for simultaneous submissions (sending to multiple places at once) as long as you let them know in your cover letter that you are doing it and then contact them immediately if your work is accepted by another journal. In general, you always want to have work in circulation. It's best to create a list of ten places that you think would be a good fit for a particular story. Send to the first five. And then when the story is rejected by one, as will most likely happen, you are ready with the next place in mind. Rejection always sends us down. Having another journal at your fingertips can help bring you back up, whereas the idea of having to research journals all over again may be enough to make you reconsider nursing school.

Keep track of where you are sending your poems, stories, and essays, either physically in a notebook or online in a document or spreadsheet. Many journals rely on submission managers as a way for writers to easily submit their work. A submission manager does not cost money, though submitting work to a journal might. One nice thing about a submission manager is that you can keep track of the progress of your work—the work has been received, the work that is in progress, the work has been declined—and it can also help you remember where you sent work to. Every journal or contest will rely on the submission manager of their choice, so you will be working across platforms. Therefore, you are in charge of keeping track of where you have submitted and where you are going to head next when the work is declined.

Submitting to literary journals used to be free. Writers were told that if an entity was charging a fee to read, then they were not to be trusted. But most literary journals, even when supported by colleges and universities, can no longer remain afloat financially without a little help from those who submit. Literary journals function with very small staffs, four or five, and most have had to move to a small submission fee to offset the numbers of submissions. Typically, a journal will charge two or three dollars. You can think of this as the money that, in the old days, you would have spent on printing and postage. Pay the fee and know it is just part of publishing.

Another route to go, aside from literary journals, is a literary contest. A contest may be hosted by a literary journal but happens only once a year. The contest often awards a monetary prize in addition to publication and the fact that your work has received a named award. Contests are more expensive, often about $25 to enter. The cost, of course, narrows the numbers of submissions, but it also quickly adds up. Sending an essay to five literary journals will, at the most, cost $15. Five contests: $125. A contest, especially a prestigious one, can be a great feather in your cap. Agents and presses may approach you when you win a contest, so winning a contest can send you on your way, but you might not be able to pay rent.

Your work will be rejected. Again and again and again. Rejection is part of the path. A major part. And you need to prepare yourself mentally. We are always filled with hope when we send work out, but then we are always sad when the work is declined. Not only will it be declined, you won't even know the reason why. No editor, or almost no editor, has time these days to send a personal note letting you know why they couldn't accept your story. A form letter will appear in your box: Sorry, this piece isn't right for us. Wish you the best in placing it.

Still, even these boilerplate rejections can actually tell you a little about how your work has been received. For example, if the language says that the story doesn't work for them and best of luck, then, for the most part you can assume the fit wasn't there. Either you misjudged their aesthetic or your aesthetic or the readiness of the story. But you can also receive a boilerplate email that says, for example, we are sorry that this piece doesn't work for us right now but please try us again. When you receive that email, you know that the fit was closer. They like your work. Note that down in your submission record. You may receive an email that encourages you to mention how much they loved your submission when you submit again. Even closer!

One day, with persistence and research, your poem or story or essay will find a home. Take the time to celebrate. Acceptances are rare. This is exciting news to be shared with your writing group or your friends. And when the work arrives in the world—its birthday—be sure to let others know through social media, email, or word of mouth. You must revel in your successes. They are few, but they are glorious.

If you send a piece of writing to ten or fifteen journals—journals that you have researched well and feel are solid fits—and the piece is resoundingly rejected, then you may decide to pull that piece from circulation and consider more revision. Put the piece in a drawer for a few months. Return, when you are ready, with fresh eyes.

Chantel Gerfen, a friend and yoga teacher, likes to think of rejection as the universe's form of protection. You thought you wanted X, but the universe knows that Y is best for you. I like to think about rejection this way because it keeps me focused on the future. When my work is declined, I may not know what I am being protected from or what is in store for me down the road, but for whatever reason, this was not the right journal, the right moment, the right essay or editor. Rejection becomes transformed into a kind of bubble that is keeping me safe until the time is right. Otherwise, rejection can make you question to your worthiness, your talents, your commitment to writing. Instead, try to let rejection be an opening to a different path or future—one that may be far better than what you thought you wanted.

PART FOUR

Void—*Bāhya kumbhaka*

50

Entering the Void

As we move toward the end of the book, it makes sense that we spend time at the bottom or end of the breath: the moment when we have exhaled all the air out of our lungs and reside in emptiness. That void has a lot to teach us even if we don't remain there long. Take some time now to return to the breath and find your three-part breath. Once again—as if for the very first time—notice the way in which the breath enters and pours *prāṇa* into the body. Let the inhalation seep into every crack and crevice; let it water all the desiccated and dried-up parts of your lungs, the places that breath rarely touches because we fail too often to breathe with intention. Just relish the inhalation for all its fullness, for the miracle that it arrives without asking, for its embodiment of joy and creation and the promise that you will always have exactly what you need (even when that might be hard to see). Then follow the exhalation down the body. Allow it to take all that no longer serves you. Feel the exhalation winnow to a point at the base of the lungs. Exhale to that point and then invite the next inhalation. Breathe like this for a few breaths, ultimately extending the inhalation to a count of four and the exhalation to a count of six. The body settles. The mind settles. Just ride the wave of each breath.

When you are ready, follow the next exhalation down to the very bottom of the lungs. Gently exhale all the air out. Don't try to drill down; rather softly sift your way to the bottom. Once you arrive, pause in emptiness. Stay here, in the void, for one or two beats. Then open yourself to the next inhalation. If you feel any grasping as you inhale, then you have tarried in the void too long. Emptying the lungs and sitting in nothingness is incredibly hard. Your body and mind will start to clutch and grab almost immediately. Remaining in the void takes practice. If you can be at the bottom with no air in or out for three or four seconds, that is amazing. Practice this breath retention every day and you will note measurable progress. Yogis add *bandhas*, or energetic locks, to this breath practice so that they can remain in emptiness for more than a minute, but I am only encouraging you to wallow for a moment in that void where nothing seems to exist. What you will find, paradoxically, is that your body is not empty but full.

This particular *prāṇāyāma*, or breath practice, is called *kumbhaka*, a word derived from the Sanskrit for pot. You are, in essence, turning your body into a pot, one that, in this case, appears empty. In yoga, it is thought that at birth each person is allocated the number of breaths they will have in this lifetime. You can never know how many breaths you have, but you can care for the breaths you have been given. Therefore, a yogi would say, if you slow your breath down, reduce the number of inhalations and exhalations, you will live longer. Many breath practices in yoga focus on slowing down the breath, taking fewer breaths, relishing what we have been given. Once again, science supports a practice passed down for 3,000 years. In general, the faster an animal breathes the shorter its lifespan. A monkey breathes thirty-two times a minute and lives on average twenty years, while elephants breathe less and live three times longer. Most humans breathe about eighteen times a minute. The intentional breathing we have been doing slows that down to ten times a minute. However, the giant tortoise breathes four times a minute and lives 300 years.

You probably won't breathe like a tortoise in this lifetime, but you can learn to linger longer at the bottom of the breath. Remember, though, that you defeat the purpose of the practice if you come out of the retention gasping for air. What you should find is that the longer you can linger in the space of emptiness, the more the space begins to pulse with something. At first, maybe you will hear your blood as it moves through your body, your pulse, maybe even your heartbeat. It is possible that each time you touch the void, you can stay a little longer, allowing yourself to explore the darkness more fully. Let the emptiness expand. In the Western world, we tend to dislike the dark. We fear what can't be seen. But almost everything that arrives in this world begins in darkness—from seeds, to babies, to stars and ideas. The darkness is the only space in our life of pure potential. Swaying in emptiness at the bottom of the breath, we are inhabiting all possibilities at once. When something comes into the light, it gets named. But the moment before it is birthed, it is only potential. And one of the only places where we can be in potential rather than actual is at the void of retention. Everything exists at that moment because nothing exists. Michael, my husband, calls this "the place where nothing takes place and everything is born."

As a writer, perhaps there is no more euphoric space to inhabit than the one where every word, every line, and every idea that has ever been said, is about to be said, or will never be said all exist at the same time. Everything that has been both accepted and exiled exists in that space. All the known and the unknown. The void brims with potential, for only in nothing can there be everything. The bottom of the breath—what we often think of as desolation, emptiness, end—is so full of possibility that there is room for nothing else. Wendell Berry has a poem entitled "To Know the Dark" and the first line reads, "To go into the dark with a light is to know the light." If you want to take the pulse of the universe before it took shape, you cannot carry the stars or a flashlight or an inhalation with you. You have to enter the dark, the void, with nothing in your hands and no air in your body. What you find, Berry assures, is that the dark, too, "blooms and sings."

51

The Alchemy of Writing

The ancients called alchemy the language of birds, a series of secret, coded processes that, when understood, could create the impossible but to anyone without understanding would appear as gibberish. The language of birds keeps me humble and reminds me that there is much in this world that I do not know, much that cannot be seen, graphed, held, counted. The world is mystical and magical and beyond our ken. Just listen to the birds. Or the whales for that matter with their laden songs traveling hundreds of miles through Homer's wine-dark sea. We can guess: mating, territorial, hunger. But we don't know. The birds have sung for millennia, and we stand outside their song. That we cannot translate the language of birds does not, then, mean the language is useless or that it doesn't exist. Rather, it points to the limits of our knowing and the riches of the unknown.

The body, our body, is rooted in the physical. We know what our senses tell us: this rock is hard; this water, wet; this garbage smells like rotten eggs. Bodily awareness begins at birth when a baby nurses minutes from the womb. We arrive embodied and remain embodied, in the same body, until the moment that we don't. To obtain a sense of how well you know your edges just close your eyes. Take your hands away from one another with pointer fingers extended. Slowly, and in darkness, move your fingers toward one another. Their tips will touch. Precisely. You know your borders, your boundaries, even when you cannot see them.

At the same time, we are made of light. As Robert Bartlett writes in his book *Real Alchemy*, "to the alchemist, everything is alive." And by everything, he means everything. Plants, animals, minerals, the chair on which you sit. Alchemists believe that all matter is pursuing perfection over eons of time. Every species in every kingdom is slowly transforming into a perfect state of balance—the perfection or oneness from which everything evolved. The alchemist assists in the process by removing any impurities and accelerating the elevation in the laboratories.

Catherine MacCoun writes in *On Becoming an Alchemist* that "the human organism, is, in and of itself, an alchemical vessel, transmuting the spiritual (pure concept) into the physical (pictures, speech, and deed)." The process of naming something is an alchemical one—casting something previously unknown (pure energy) into language (form). One day, Covid-19 doesn't exist. Then it does. That is alchemy. Before there was nothing; then there is something. For the alchemist, that act of thinking or naming—where concept or pure consciousness or energy becomes solidified into word—is a downward movement toward matter and away from light. It is a movement toward heaviness. As I wrote earlier, words become concrete and inflexible. They lose both levity and mobility. The known, then, becomes a kind of burden: what is birthed must be carried.

For the alchemist, the heaviness and inflexibility of matter is not a bad thing. It is sought. This is such an important point for writers and artists in general. MacCoun writes, "In alchemy, the nearest thing to an ideal state is an ongoing state of disarray." In other words, the more messy, the more ideal. While many religious traditions would suggest that the sins of the world come from the body's needs and desires and, therefore, need to be either rejected or transcended, both yoga and alchemy start with the physical world as the very medium for transformation. We don't reject the ugly, the difficult, the sinful, the messy, the vexed; rather we see them as the best possible places to begin our work because they provide the greatest possibility for transformation. The uglier, the better.

The manifest as well as all the words we use to describe the manifest exist on the horizontal, so we begin there—both in terms of writing and in terms of becoming better human beings. In alchemy, this is the dark, sticky, heavy matter that holds all the possibility of becoming gold. Whether in relation to ourselves, our speakers, our characters, or the act of writing itself, if there is no mess then there is no room for transformation. When you are struggling and flailing and wandering about the house asking why you ever thought you were born to write, you are at the black stage of the alchemical process: putrefaction, decay.

Alchemists first allow for rot. They create containers in their laboratories not to just hold but to *incubate* decay. They are tender toward their mess, tender for the long haul, because decay can happen over the course of years. Alchemists rush nothing. Anne Lamott calls rot a "shitty first draft." I have heard other writers refer to this initial phase as the word vomit. Alchemists call this phase the Black Phase or Nigredo and it is by far the longest and most tortuous part of the process. The substance at hand must suffer, which, in writing, means both you and your draft. More to the point, you cannot begin anywhere except in decay and rot. Alchemists cannot skip steps. Death and loss must occur before something new can arise.

Alchemists are involuting from form back to energy. They are helping the universe return to oneness, just like the yogis. In essence, artists work the same way. Artists use the things of the world—words, paint, clay—to move from the horizontal to the vertical—from the subject of a poem, story, or essay toward the "so what." Monet is not really painting a haystack; he is painting light. The alchemist and the writer move into the next phase of the process, involute closer to energy, when they begin to separate the matter before them into its essential elements. For the alchemist, this means separating a substance, in the lab, into mercury, sulfur, and salt (not actual mercury, sulfur, and salt but the substance's spirit, fire, and body). For the writer, this means coming to understand what it is that you are trying to say. You sit with the mess long enough that you begin to see the shape of what it is you are making. In alchemy, this is the White Phase, a period marked by fire and calcination. Burning. Whether a poem in its becoming or the leaves of lemon balm fermenting, the excess burns away so that only the bone remains. You must destroy in order to create.

In the final phase, the Red Phase, a new substance is born when its exalted elements are recombined. Your draft, your self, or your lemon balm have been fully purified, no dross remains. In alchemy, at the moment of recombination, the substance, an elixir for example, receives a new birth chart. Through separation, purification, and recombination, the alchemist isolates a substance into its most pure and essential aspects and then brings those purified essentials together again to create gold. They involute something dark and heavy back toward its essential nature as light and energy. Writing works the same way. We begin with words that are heavy and fixed and burn them to their most essential. Then we dissolve them in the waters of metaphor and imagery so that something new is born, something that has not existed before, something that moves and changes and transforms with every reading, something less like matter and more like light.

One more word about alchemy. What separates alchemy from science is not the process but rather the intention. Unlike traditional scientists who consider their materials dead, the alchemists know their materials have lifeforce energy and consciousness. An alchemist begins with the premise that everything in the world is energy; it's all the same thing. Robert Bartlett writes in *Real Alchemy*, "the alchemist becomes an ingredient in [their] own experiment." They are no different from the substance in the crucible. This means that when an alchemist works, their own transformation is as important as the transformation of the substance. Medieval alchemists had an *oratorium* in their labs, a separate space where they could meditate and pray alongside the journey of their substance. When their substance was facing its mortification, the alchemist also traveled through a dark night of the soul. They sympathized with their materials and believed their consciousness or intention could change the outcome. Quantum physics bears this out.

Our writing transforms us. We sympathize with our drafts, our characters, and our attempt to articulate what is internal, unformed, and unnamed in ourselves. The writing process does not occur outside of us. We transmute with our characters. In finding their humanity and complexity, we develop more compassion, move closer toward our essential nature as light. You cannot subject yourself to mess day after day, burn the dead, hold bone in your hand, and not see a haystack as a container of light. The mess becomes clarified, if only for a moment, in art. We see reality, even if what we see is still painful. It's a clean pain, distilled and pure.

Which is why it doesn't matter if anyone ever reads what you write, if your work is published, if you have 10,000 followers on Instagram, because the work is what matters. Every day that you sit down with your mess, every day you burn the dross, every day that you bring together the purified and essential so that they become something greater than they were before you worked with them is a day you step closer to your own essential nature, a day you step closer to becoming the light that you are. Nothing in the writing process or the alchemical process is easy or free. There is burning and fermenting and the destruction of the ego. Ultimately, MacCoun writes, the alchemist becomes the sun that radiates forever outward, "giving away every last bit of itself." Nothing is kept. All is given. To return to the rainbow at the very start of this book, we want to be in the world knowing that we already have everything that we need. Fullness is full. The rainbow is always there. From that place, we can give because fullness still remains.

52

Surrender Ritual

As writers, we offer. That is all we can do. We cannot control the reception of our words any more than we can control the flight of birds. Michael and I remind each other constantly that art is service to the world. *Karma* yoga is the yoga of selfless service. You act and then you release all expectations. A brief story I carry with me is an Indian one I read long ago. A crow lands on a coconut high up in a tree. As the crow lands, the coconut falls to the ground. The crow can never know if it caused the coconut to fall or if it was time for the coconut to fall. In the same way, we offer and then we let go of results. This means that when our work goes out into the world and is rejected, we cannot claim that we are bad writers. Nor, if it is accepted, can we own the acclaim either. Sometimes the work lands in one place, sometimes another. Coconuts fall. That's about all that can be said.

You can claim neither your successes nor your failures as your own. You do not own them. They are not yours. You simply offer and then you return to your writing.

This is a hard lesson to learn—both in times of sadness and joy. When we feel our writing is going poorly, we so easily blame ourselves or blame others or blame anything. But such energy is surely wasted. Who should the coconut blame? Or the crow? Each can only be responsible for their specific action. And then, harder, if we do experience success, we must check our ego. That is not ours to own either. Yes, we have worked hard. Yes, we are dedicated. But "success" is just as impossible to track as failure. Who is the "you" who just published that story? Is it separate from the teachers who mentored you, or the writers who inspired you, or the writing group that carried you, or the parents who bore you, or the thousands upon thousands of generations who remained alive long enough to produce offspring? How much is yours to claim? Again, you only offer. Be grateful in joy and in suffering, grateful to those in your life who make it possible for you to experience both.

I leave you with a final ritual that reminds us all to remain humble and to remember that we cannot own what happens with our words. If the ritual speaks to you, then I would encourage you to practice it often. The origins are with Sri Sri Anandamurti's *guru puja*; I have modified it here to make it more accessible.

Begin in a seated posture and with your breath. Cup your hands before your heart, making a bowl. Imagine filling the bowl with a single worry or a single joy. Perhaps you imagine placing the draft of your poem in your bowl or maybe the award you recently received. Perhaps it is your father's dementia that you need to place in the bowl or your worry over repairs needed for your car. Big or small. Some days it will be a joy that goes in the bowl, something for which you are grateful, and some days a sorrow. Hold the bowl at your heart and feel whatever the feeling is that arises. Let the feeling work its way into your flesh and bones, the cavities and capillaries of your body. Let your heart ache or expand. Give the feeling qualities—is it dark, dull, tarry, and black (*tamasic*); fire-filled and raging like anger or jealousy (*rajasic*); or full of joy and light (*sattvic*)? Feel it for as long as you can. Name it. Sadness, I feel you. Heartache, I feel you. Rapture, I feel you. Then, when you are ready, take yourself belly down to the ground. In yoga, this is called full *pranam*. Belly to the earth, arms stretched overhead, still holding the bowl, face down. You cannot be any lower to the ground. You are earth. Release your cup and let its contents go. Stay there. Feel your heart beat. When you rise, take nothing with you. Start again.

Conclusion

For one last time, close your eyes. Notice that because of your daily practice, when you turn your gaze inward and locate your breath, you return home. Stillness becomes the familiar, and the harried pace of the world outside the breath becomes the exception. You may spend more time outside the breath, but you now recognize that those long inhalations and long exhalations are where you want to spend your day, your life. Reside in the hammock of your breath.

The breath is seasonal. Every complete inhalation and exhalation teaches us about rebirth, starting over, the promise that, no matter how many times you fall or falter, you, like the crocus in the spring, will rise again. Once you have found your long four- and six-count breath and have allowed the quiet to permeate every cell in your body so that your whole body has been touched by the awareness of consciousness, return once again to inhalation. This time, as you inhale, imagine taking the inhalation up the front of the body. Feel it grow from the base of the lungs to the shore of the collarbones. This is spring. Imagine, then, the summer of the breath passing over the top of the body. This pause will be shorter because, while summer is all about fullness, summer also has an intensity that cannot be born for long periods. It's too hot. Let the season of summer float across the top of your body as you hold fullness inside for just a moment. Now, exhale down the back of the body, the long slow slide of fall. Just like the leaves instruct, autumn is the season of letting go. No leaf sifts to the ground in struggle. It releases and then glides to the earth. Feel the surrender of the season, as well as its length, as you exhale down the back of the body. At the bottom of the exhalation, meet winter and void. Bare-limbed branches in elemental outline against gray sky. Glide across the bottom of the body and the breath. Winter, like summer, is no place to linger. These extremes in the seasons are best experienced for shorter amounts of time. Welcome winter into the breath and the lesson it teaches of embracing the dark, but you need not stay long. Just a moment. Inhale again and bring your body into spring.

Practiced this way, the breath makes a circle or square. Up the front, over the collarbones, down the back, across the base of the pelvis, back up. Be present for each season and what the seasons teach us about being in the world. Every breath is a year. Likewise, each season of the year is associated with part of the breath. Such awareness, then, allows you to be fully present to the fullness of summer and to know the intense heat of August will not last, nor will dark January mornings. Not unlike eating seasonally, breathing seasonally puts us back in touch with the human bodies of our ancestors, who only a short time ago could not afford to live anywhere other than the present moment. Breathing seasonally also helps with a rejection from a magazine or a day where the writing goes less than well. You are in late fall, early winter. Wait for the next inhalation and allow the process to begin again.

Breathe this way for as long as feels good. Let the seasons turn in your body. Let spring unfold into summer and fall winnow down to winter. Feel fullness, feel void, and feel the transitions that bring us in and out of both. Notice that the breath never stops, nor does time. Even the present moment is an always moving present. We do not step out of time. We do not step out of the breath. And we do not step out of the fact that we were born to write. Writing moves like our breath, from earth to sky and back again, always a process, always a miracle.

BIBLIOGRAPHY

Adele, Deborah. *The Yamas and the Niyamas: Exploring Yoga's Ethical Practices*. Duluth MN: On-Word Bound Books, 2009.

Bartlett, Robert Allen. *Real Alchemy: A Primer of Practical Alchemy*. Lake Worth FL: Ibis Press, 2009.

Bell, Madison Smartt. *Narrative Design: Working with Imagination, Craft, and Form*. New York: Norton, 1997.

Berry, Wendell. *The Selected Poems of Wendell Berry*. Berkely, CA: Counterpoint, 1999.

Berthoff, Ann. "Recognition, Representation, and Revision." *The Journal of Basic Writing* 3, no. 1 (1981): 19–32.

The Bhagavad Gītā. Trans. Eknath Easwaran. Canada: Nilgiri Press, 2007.

Blondin, Sarah. *Heart Minded: How to Hold Yourself and Others in Love*. Boulder, CO: Sounds True, 2020.

Burdick, Alan. "Why Nouns Slow Us Down, and Why Linguistics Might Be in a Bubble." *The New Yorker*. May 15, 2018. Available online: https://www.newyorker.com/science/lab-notes/why-nouns-slow-us-down-and-why-linguistics-might-be-in-a-bubble (accessed January 23, 2023).

Burroway, Janet. *Writing Fiction: A Guide to Narrative Craft*. Eighth edition. Boston: Longman, 2011.

Cameron, Julia. *The Artist's Way: A Spiritual Path to Higher Creativity*. New York: Tarcher/Putnam, 1992.

Caron, Amber. Personal correspondence. Spring 2022.

Chavez, Felicia Rose. *The Anti-Racist Writing Workshop: How to Decolonize the Creative Writing Classroom*. Chicago: Haymarket Books, 2021.

Clark, Bernie. Yin Yoga Teacher Training. Spring 2021.

Clark, Roy Peter. *Writing Tools. 50 Essential Strategies for Every Writer*. New York: Little Brown, 2006.

Cott, Jonathan. *Dinner with Lenny: The Long Lost Interview with Leonard Bernstein*. New York: Oxford University Press, 2013.

Csikszentmihalyi, Mihaly. *Flow: The Psychology of Optimal Experience*. Harper Perennial Modern Classics. New York: Harper, 2008.

De Mille, Agnes. *Martha: The Life and Work of Martha Graham: A Biography*. New York: Random House, 1991.

Dillard, Annie. *The Writing Life*. New York: Harper & Row, 1989.

Doerr, Anthony. *Cloud Cuckoo Land*. New York: Scribner, 2021.

Doyle, Brian. "Leap." In *Leaping: Revelations and Epiphanies*. Chicago: Loyola Press, 2003.

Fadiman, Anne. *Ex Libris: Confessions of a Common Reader*. New York: Farrar, Straus & Giroux, 2000.

Gardner, John. *The Art of Fiction: Notes on Craft for Young Writers*. New York: Vintage Books, 1991.

Gardner, John. *On Moral Fiction*. New York: Basic Books, 1978.

Gerard, Philip. *Creative Nonfiction: Researching and Crafting Stories of Real Life*. Cincinnati, OH: Story Free Press, 1996.

Gonzalez, Christopher. Personal correspondence. January 20, 2022.

Gordon, Mary. "Moral Fiction." *The Atlantic*. 2005 Fiction Issue. Available online: https://www.theatlantic.com/magazine/archive/2005/08/moral-fiction/304128/ (accessed January 21, 2023).

Greenough, Sarah. Ed. *My Far Away One: Selected Letters of Georgia O'Keeffe and Alfred Stieglitz, Volume One 1915–1933*. New Haven CT: Yale University Press, 2011.

Gwartney, Debra. "Cake." *Brevity*. Issue 47. September 2014. Available online: https://brevitymag.com/nonfiction/cake/ (accessed January 23, 2023).

Huber, Sonya. "The Three Words That Almost Ruined Me as a Writer: 'Show, Don't Tell.'" *Literary Hub*. September 27, 2019. Available online: https://lithub.com/the-three-words-that-almost-ruined-me-as-a-writer-show-dont-tell/ (accessed January 22, 2023).

Iyengar, B.K.S. *Light on Yoga*. Revised edition. New York: Schocken Books, 1979.

Jones, Edward P. "The First Day." In *Lost in the City*. 20th anniversary edition. New York: Amistad, 2012.

The Kabir Book: Forty-Four of the Ecstatic Poems of Kabir. Trans. Robert Bly. Boston: Beacon Press, 1977.

Kean, Sam. *Caesar's Last Breath: Decoding the Secrets of the Air around Us*. New York: Little Brown, 2017.

Kerouac, Jack. "Essentials of Spontaneous Prose." Available online: https://writing.upenn.edu/~afilreis/88v/kerouac-spontaneous.html (accessed January 22, 2023).

Kimmerer, Robin Wall. *Braiding Sweetgrass: Indigenous Wisdom, Scientific Knowledge, and the Teachings of Plants*. Minneapolis MN: Milkweed Editions, 2015.

King, Stephen. *On Writing Well: A Memoir of the Craft*. New York: Pocket Books, 2000.

Ladinsky, Daniel. *A Year with Hafiz: Daily Contemplations*. New York: Penguin, 2011.

Lahiri, Jhumpa. "Mrs. Sen's." In *Interpreter of Maladies*. Boston: Houghton Mifflin, 1999: 111–35.

Lakoff, George and Mark Johnson. *Metaphors We Live By*. Chicago: University of Chicago Press, 2003.

Lamott, Anne. *Bird by Bird: Some Instructions on Writing and Life*. New York: Anchor Books, 1995.

Lorde, Audre. *The Selected Works of Audre Lorde*. Ed. Roxane Gay. New York: Norton, 2020.

MacCoun, Catherine. *On Becoming an Alchemist: A Guide for the Modern Magician*. Boulder, CO: Trumpeter Books, 2008.

Menakem, Resmaa. *My Grandmother's Hands: Racialized Trauma and the Pathway to Mending Our Hearts and Bodies*. Las Vegas NV: Central Recovery Press, 2017.

Miller, Brenda. "A Braided Heart: Shaping the Lyric Essay." In *Writing Creative Nonfiction*. Ed. Philip Gerard. 14–24. Cincinnati OH: Writer's Digest Books, 2001.
Moore, Dinty W. *The Truth of the Matter: Art and Craft in Creative Nonfiction*. New York: Pearson, 2007.
Morrison, Toni. *Paradise*. New York: Plume Books, 1999.
Nabokov, Vladimir. *Speak, Memory*. First Vintage International edition. New York: Vintage International, 1989.
Nhat Hanh, Thich. *The World We Have: A Buddhist Approach to Peace and Ecology*. Berkeley, CA: Parallax Press, 2004.
O'Connor, Flannery. *Mystery and Manners: Occasional Prose*. First paperback edition. New York: Farrar, Straus, & Giroux, 1970.
Oliver, Mary. *The House of Light*. Boston: Beacon Press, 1992.
Patanjali. *The Yoga Sutras of Patanjali*. Trans. Sri Swami Satchidananda. Third edition. Buckingham, VA: Integral Yoga Publications, 2014.
Ramakrishna. *The Gospel of Sri Ramakrishna*. Trans. Swami Nikhilananda. Abridged edition. Third edition. New York: Ramakrishna-Vivekananda Center, 1974.
Ray, Annie Pringle. Manuscript diary, 1881–1884. Author's collection.
Rekdal, Paisley. Radio Interview. "Utah Poet Laureate Paisley Rekdal: A New Collection and the Old Railroad." KUER. May 7, 2019.
Rilke, Rainer Maria. *Letters to a Young Poet*. Merchant Books, 2012.
Roche, Lorin. *The Radiance Sutras: 112 Gateways to the Yoga of Wonder and Delight*. Boulder CO: Sounds True, 2014.
Romano, Tom. *Blending Genre, Altering Genre: Writing Multigenre Papers*. Portsmouth NH: Heinemann, 2000.
Roorbach, Bill. *Writing Life Stories: How to Make Memories into Memoirs, Ideas into Essays, and Life into Literature*. Cincinnati, OH: Writer's Digest Books, 2008.
Sadhguru. *Inner Engineering: A Yogi's Guide to Joy*. New York: Spiegel and Grau, 2016.
Shumaker, Peggy. *Just Breathe Normally*. Lincoln, NE: University of Nebraska Press, 2007.
Stoppard, Tom. *The Real Thing*. Reprinted with revisions. London: Faber & Faber, 1983.
Sukrungruang, Ira. "To Disappear & To Find." *Brevity*. Issue 66. January 2022. Available online: https://brevitymag.com/nonfiction/to-disappear/ (accessed January 22, 2023).
Svātmārāma. *The Haṭha Yoga Pradīpika*. Trans. Brian Dana Akers. Woodstock, NY: YogaVidya, 2002.
Towles, Amor. "Amor Towles on Bringing a Historical Setting to Life." *Literary Hub*. February 4, 2022. Available online: https://lithub.com/amor-towles-on-bringing-a-historical-setting-to-life/ (accessed January 22, 2023).
Trungpa, Chogyam Rinpoche. "The Decision to Become a Buddhist." *Lion's Roar*. May 16, 2017. Available online: https://www.lionsroar.com/the-decision-to-become-a-buddhist/ (accessed on January 27, 2023).
The Upanishads. Trans. Eknath Easwaran. Canada: Nilgiri Press, 2007.
Van der Kolk, Bessel. *The Body Keeps the Score: Brain, Mind, and the Body in the Trauma of Healing*. New York: Penguin, 2014.

Van Meter, Ryan. "First." In *If You Knew Then What I Know Now*. Louisville KY: Sarabande Books, 2011.

Woolf, Virginia. *A Room of One's Own*. First Harvest edition. New York: Harvest Books, 1989.

Woolf, Virginia. "A Sketch of the Past." In *Moments of Being*. Second edition. New York: Harvest Books, 1985.

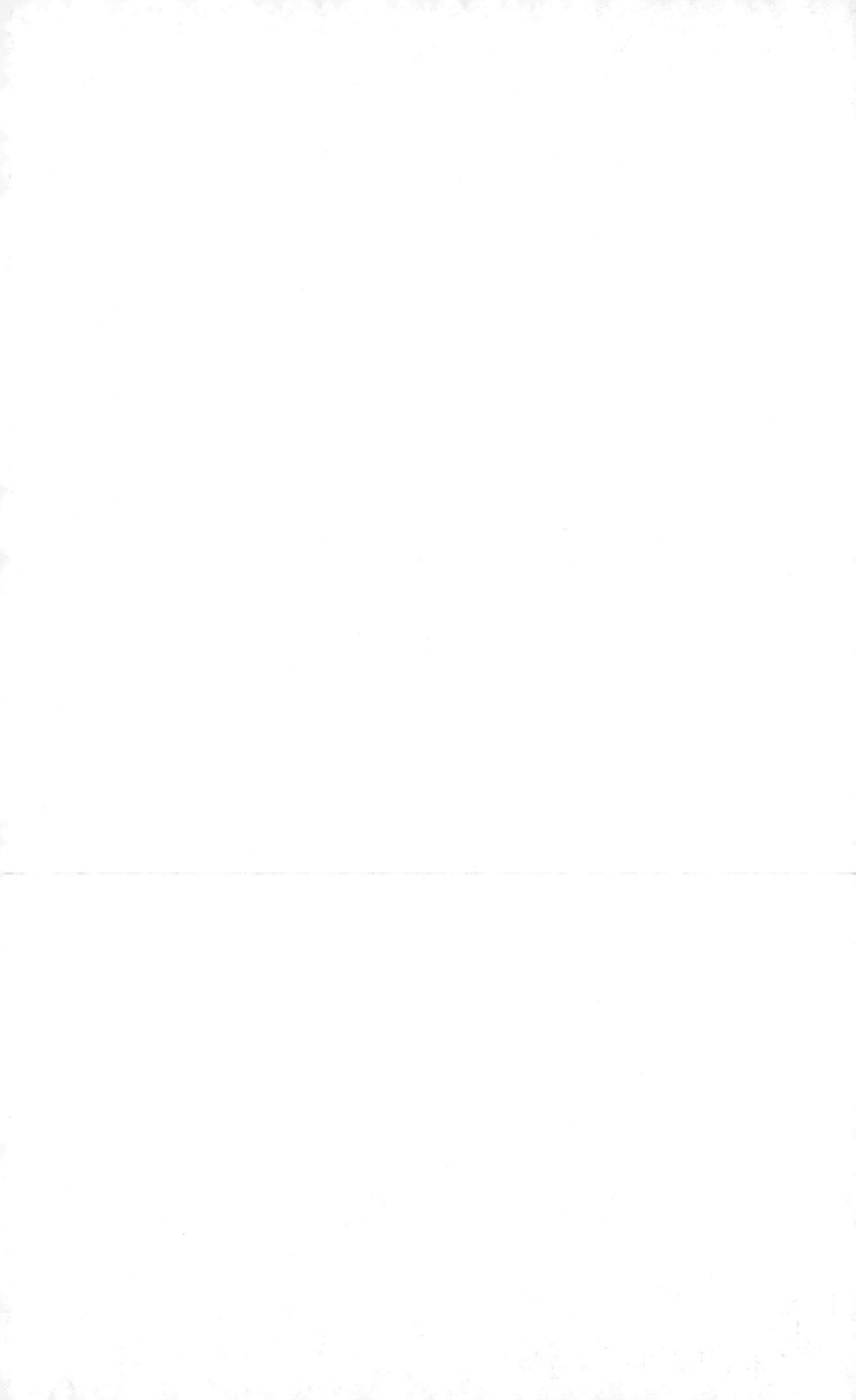

www.ingramcontent.com/pod-product-compliance
Lightning Source LLC
Chambersburg PA
CBHW071843230426
43671CB00012B/2057